I0442080

Forever Young, Forever Fit

Nik Helbig

Disclaimer:

The health and fitness information presented in this book is intended as an educational resource. It is not substitute for medical advice. Consult a healthcare professional before performing exercises or any activities provided in this book, particularly if you are pregnant or have known health and mental health issues. Discontinue any activity if you suffer pain or discomfort. Author, publisher and distributors of such information make no warranty and take no responsibility of any kind in regard to the content of the information presented in this book.

DEDICATION

To Oliver Helbig

Table of Contents

"You can't help getting older, but you don't have to get old."
George Burns

Introduction

The original version of this book was written just for me. It was a personal sketchbook of facts, articles, and philosophy on the subject of living well—really well.

It seems to me such a waste to spend one's life building up wisdom and relationships, only to languish in later years, becoming a burden to those we care about. It could be because I saw my own grandmother deteriorate with no apparent cause. She was only fifty-eight, but she had lost interest in life, deciding she was old and hopeless. My parents said then that that is how it is going to be for the family because we share the same "genes."

Then I witnessed other people's grandparents and parents. The reality was different. I felt the unfairness.

I majored in biochemistry and physiology in the university, basically to understand genes and—among other things—to find evidence of a God.

While the God question is beyond the scope of this book, I realized that a lot of my family's gene issue was really a product of poor lifestyle choices. We were fatter and clumsier than others in the community then. My father, who had the idea that studies for good grades were paramount, never allowed us time for sports. He had never done sports himself. We never did anything outside our crammed three-bedroom apartment.

Now that I am an adult, I see my parents and even siblings withering away just like the generation before them. Genes. Or is it not?

I struggled with obesity, chronic illnesses, allergies, and depression for decades. Exercise to me meant hours of obsessive running. Diet meant anorexia.

When I stopped the running and anorexia—with thanks to friends who cared—the weight piled back on. The constant battle with food and exercise went on.

What a waste of life it was to keep being preoccupied with stuff like this.

I met my in-laws in my thirties. They are the polar opposite of my parents. At the time of writing this book, my grandmother-in-law, ninety-four, whom we call Omi, still lives independently in an apartment. My parents-in-law live up in a mountain in Austria, which has a harsh environment compared to comfy Singapore, where my parents live. They are fiercely self-preserving, stay physically active, and are today much younger in physical state than my own parents, who, now in their seventies, have problems taking only a few steps.

Living healthy has a whole lot to do with one's mental state. The only difference between my parents and my in-laws is their attitude toward health and aging.

You might ask why I wasn't able to coax my own family into healthier living. There is such a thing as a black sheep, the prophet who is rejected in his own town. This is the reason why St. Francis of Assisi had to go talk to little creatures.

In many ways, you, the reader, are my version of St. Francis's "little creatures." I have collected a valuable trove of information. These are ten immutable laws

- to stay healthy, fit, and viable for as long as life allows;
- to make the best of our time on this earth; and
- to enable us to be there for our loved ones, our society, and ourselves so we may enjoy living well.

There is so much we can do when we're truly alive. My wish—and I guess that of every other person on this planet—is to live as long and as abundantly as possible for as long as we can help it.

This book is dedicated to everyone who is searching for the truth behind staying healthy and fit for life. I am simply sharing the facts I have put together after two decades of thought, research, the observation of people across continents, and self-experimentation.

Authors have written many books on the subjects of health, fitness, and anti-aging. No other books are like mine. The limitations of those books lie in the following facts:

- Diet books written by dieticians tell us that diet is the key.
- Fitness books written by fitness pros imply that exercise is the answer.
- Medical books written by doctors imply that aging is a natural process.
- Metaphysical books written by philosophers tend to get the biochemistry wrong.
- Other books tend to be centered on managing aging rather than obliterating the effects of aging altogether.
- E-books found on the Internet can be useful, but many are health supplement catalogs in disguise.

Keeping young and fit is multifaceted and requires a lifestyle revamp. This requires work in many aspects of life, not just focusing on one or two narrow subjects.

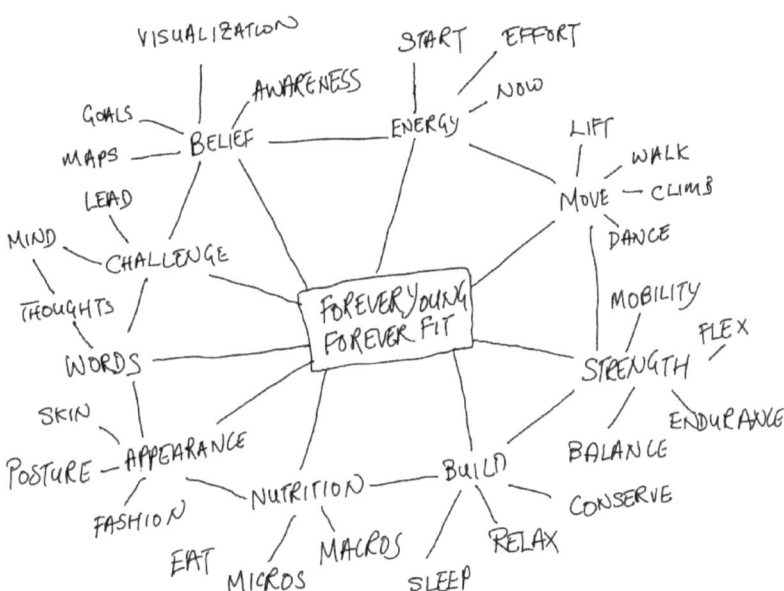

Everything is Connected

There are close connections among environment, body, and mind.
It is often better to be moderately proficient at every aspect of our lives than to be master of one while neglecting others. Being extreme in anything undermines the reason why we do that thing in the first place.

An avid runner thinks he or she is running to keep fit, but the runner ends up wearing out joints, losing skin, and suffering poor posture due to bone loss. An avid dieter becomes vegetarian in an effort to be healthy, but he or she only ends up having weak muscles, becoming prone to falls, and being stressed out. A wealthy businessman earns himself a wealthy lifestyle but ages due to stress at work.

The road to staying young and healthy is having a balanced life. But what is balance? What do we really need to balance?

Balance is not simply about doing things moderately, nor is it about doing something more intensely or less intensely. We're not referring to balancing a seesaw, which moves on only one plane.

The balance required to stay young and fit is like spinning a plate on a stick. To find balance, one must keep many directions of force in equilibrium. While focusing on exercise, dieting, and work is good, one must also commit to other lifestyle practices.

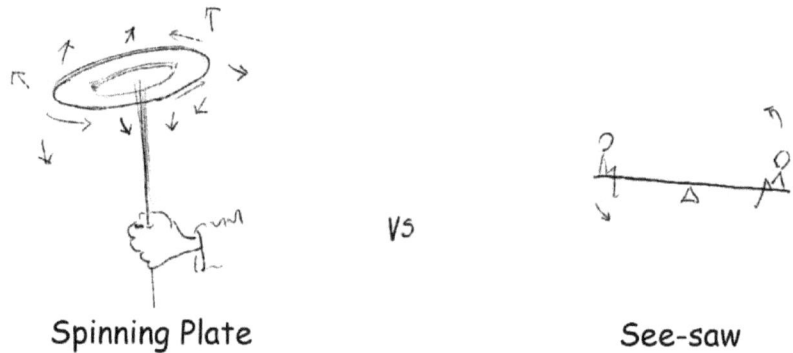

Spinning Plate   VS   See-saw

The chapters in this book will, as thoroughly as possible, elaborate on the things we need to work on to make certain lifestyle changes necessary to stay young and fit. I will present the information in a way so any busy person can find the relevant information quickly without pouring through tedious facts and research material. Literature for extra reading will be available in lists on our website. For those who have deeper interests in some of the subjects, there will be abundant material.

The Age Box

How often do we hear people say, "She looks young for her age"? More often than not, this kind of comment is targeted at someone who is middle aged or older.

If someone came up to you and said, "You look young for your age," would you consider this a compliment? Perhaps, but what does this statement really mean?

It means that all people should look a certain way as they reach a certain age.

That is complete nonsense, of course. We all develop differently. Some of us know how to keep youthful, while some of us just let ourselves go.

Society sets its sights very low. The bulk of people in society actually look worse and age faster than they should. There is a reason for this, which we will discuss in the next chapter.

Herd instinct takes over. We create "age boxes." We tell ourselves there is a certain way to look at a certain age. We put others in their age boxes, and in so doing we put ourselves in a box too.

Once we're in the age box, our minds gets trapped. We're made to believe that getting old with time is inevitable. Even if we're one of the few who knows how to keep himself or herself youthful, something will tell us we're "above the average." This thinking doesn't help since there is a tendency for us to believe that the norm is deterioration with age.

We will mention this age box again in some chapters of this book. This will help us be even more aware of it. Awareness will release us from this mind trap.

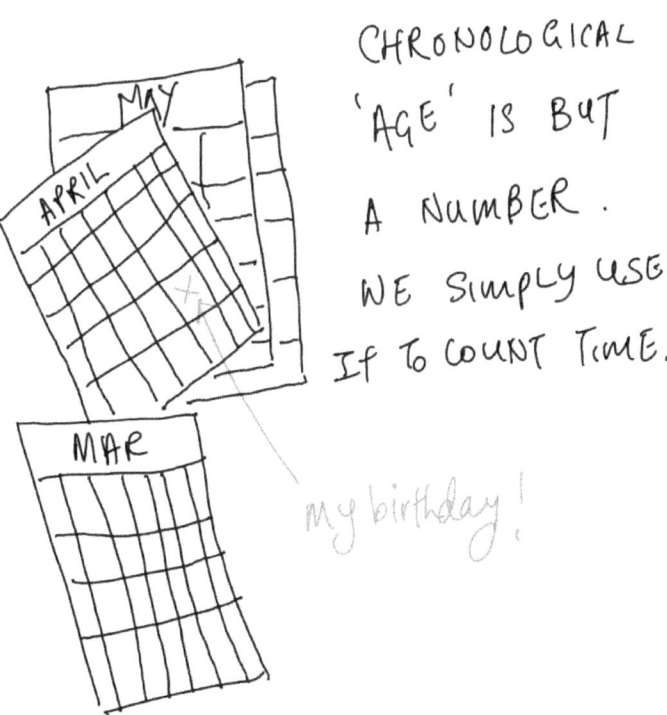

CHRONOLOGICAL 'AGE' IS BUT A NUMBER. WE SIMPLY USE IT TO COUNT TIME.

my birthday!

What is Your Actual Age?

To describe how many years we have lived from birth, we use the word *age*. Age is really only a number we use to count time. This time, which we count, is our chronological age. Apart from that number, or the number of candles on our birthday cakes, there should be nothing significant about our chronological age—unless we choose to make it so.

We know this to be true by observing groups of people of different ages. A group of seven-year-olds, for example, all look and move like seven-year-olds. As kids we all look the same age as our friends in class.

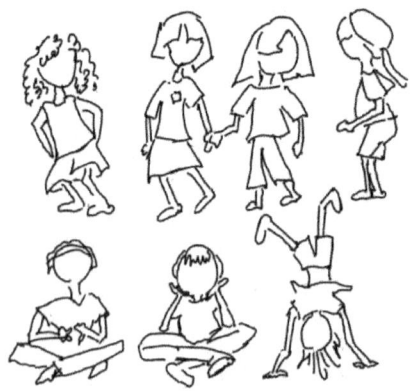

Seventeen-year-olds within a group may have different builds, but physiologically they are similar. As teens we begin to mature at different rates, but we still have the resemblance of standard teenagers.

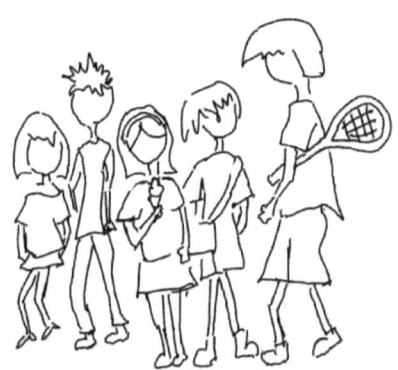

By age thirty, people start to age differently. By adulthood, people of the same age look less and less consistent within a particular age group.

In middle age and beyond, individuals from one age-group can look decades different from each other. The older they get, the more physical abilities vary.

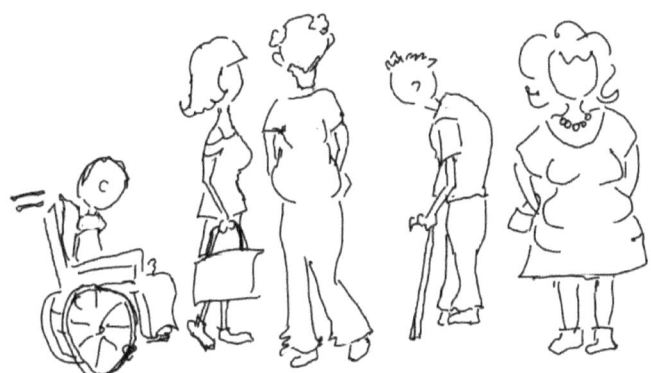

Genetically, we don't differ very much from our peers. During childhood, before time and events get a chance to take control of our lives, we all look practically the same. In our teen years we even mature around the same time.

Our environment and lifestyle largely affect what differentiates us physiologically.

During our prime adult years, we unwittingly do something to ourselves to create this change. Some of us keep good form and function while others just lose it.

This doesn't happen overnight. The aging process starts early on. It happens so gradually that we don't realize it till the change becomes obvious.

The great majority of us get old before we really should. Why? This is because it takes a whole lot more energy to preserve our youthfulness than it takes to do nothing and get old. It is natural human behavior to go the way of least effort.

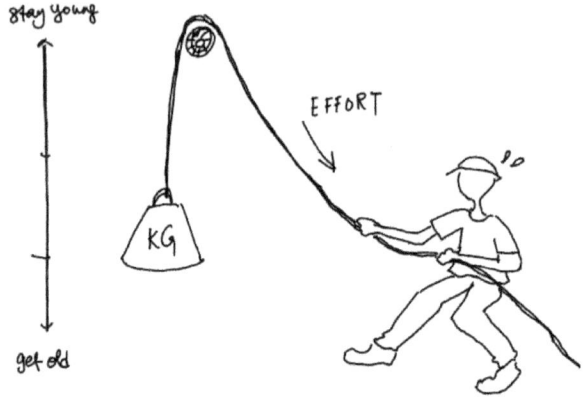

There is no effortless solution to keeping young and fit. Halting the degeneration of aging requires effort, but it gets easier to do if you keep at it.

Real Age is Only Partially Related to Your Physical Health.

During routine medical examinations, doctors measure health according to the usual parameters:

- Blood pressure
- ECG
- Blood cholesterol
- Cancer screening
- Bone-density checks
- Blood sugar
- Body weight

These parameters give an idea whether our bodies are at risk for the following ailments:

- Hypertension
- Heart disease
- Stroke, heart attack, or blood-vessel blockage
- Cancer
- Osteoporosis
- Arthritis

- Diabetes

- Obesity

Incidentally, these diseases are chronic in nature and caused by poor lifestyle habits; these conditions are rarely of the acute nature, which means they don't kill quickly. Chronic diseases don't happen suddenly or occur from one day to the next; they manifest themselves gradually over decades. Nor are these of the infectious kind.

If you pass each medical test from the doctor, you get a clean bill of health. This indicates only that you're not sick. Being given the label "not sick" doesn't mean anything today if your lifestyle will lead you to ill health tomorrow.

Chronic diseases like those listed above develop over time. Each takes decades for the symptoms to show up in the individual. We observe these ailments more commonly in the older population. People don't get ill because they are old. They get ill when they are old because they started the process when they were young. The initiation phase of these diseases occurred decades earlier. Younger adults who adopt poor lifestyle habits may not suffer the symptoms of these illnesses, but these illnesses have already taken root. Unless lifestyle changes are made early, diseases will just progress until they become noticeable in medical tests. We contract these illnesses early on in life unawares. Most life-threatening illnesses today are really self-inflicted.

Chronic illness is an unnecessary scourge of aging. Without illness, there are little "signs of aging" to begin with.

No doubt symptoms of many illnesses today can be alleviated with drugs. One can live on a cocktail of pills, stents, and dialysis—or have multiple surgeries. The result will often be a compromised life.

The only solution is a holistic lifestyle change as early on in life as possible. While it is never too late to start, doing it now is paramount.

We Have Evolved to Age

We cannot live forever, and yes, our bodies are programmed to change with time. There are things we cannot do anything about, such as our genetics, the environment, and living conditions. There is, however, enough information out there to understand the process of aging. We know the causes, and there is so much we can do for ourselves to put aging out of our lives. We can live fully forever to the end.

It is the stuff we can work on that is most effective in solving the most acute problems of aging. This, however, demands a permanent lifestyle change.

In this book I will highlight factors that cause people to get old. And I will address actions we can all take to slow down or even halt the aging process. There are things all of us can do holistically to change the course of our lives forever. These concepts represent a web of interconnected lifestyle laws, which are immutable.

Chapter 1: The Power of Belief

Consider yourself embarking on a journey for the rest of your life. This is the journey of a new lifestyle. This lifestyle requires your full attention, awareness, discipline, and motivation. You will reap rewards the moment you begin the journey, which will become second nature to those who stick with it and make it part of their lives.

By then you will see a transformation in your physical self. Others will not only notice your energy and good physique but also wonder about your ability to stay in such great shape with seemingly little effort.

Before you can even start, you need to believe that change is necessary. You have to make changes, and these changes will bring results. These results are worth every amount of effort and time you put in. You buy yourself decades of a better life.

You have to believe you can do it. Belief is the beginning of every successful venture. Harness the power to believe that you can get forever young and forever fit. Here's a story:

Two groups of kids were sent to a park to look for Easter eggs. One group was told there were five eggs hidden on the grounds, while the other group was told that the Easter bunny had left hundreds of eggs behind and that they needed to collect as many as possible.

Time passed, and the first group of kids returned very quickly with five eggs.

The second group didn't come back until the teacher called them in. That group returned with dozens of eggs in their basket.

Whether you get five eggs or dozens depends on how many eggs you believe you can get in the first place.

To achieve your goal of a younger, fitter you, you first have to believe a younger, fitter version of yourself is just waiting to emerge.

Believe in Yourself

We believe in many things. Some of these things are concepts that cannot even be proven to exist. Yet we believe them with all our hearts. If you're able to believe in the loads of stuff you cannot see, feel, or even understand, you can believe in yourself.

Believe that you have the ability to accomplish whatever it is you set out to do. That is all you need to get started. You don't need the blessings of other people to get started. It would be nice to have support, especially from your loved ones, but that is not necessary.

No one needs to believe in you except you.

Believe you can get forever young, forever fit. You can if you take the journey mapped out in this book. Along the way, you will see improvements in your body. You will find in yourself the motivation to make continuous changes to your lifestyle. You will see changes looking back at you in the mirror. Others will notice the new you too.

Ultimately, that is the goal set out for you in this book.

Aging is Optional

Human beings are the only creatures on this planet who understand the concept of aging and death. Animals don't know their life is temporary; they don't understand what it means to get old. If you have kept a pet, you will realize that even an old dog or cat behaves like a young animal…until he or she falls sick or has to slow down or dies. Animals don't age. They simply live to live then they die.

We're different. We set timetables for ourselves to get old. When we lose track of things, get weak, get sick, and lose our senses, we assume this is the natural course of things. Since it is expected of us to go like that, we don't think it is necessary to do anything about it.

The truth is that we have to.

Thanks to scientific developments, we're living longer. Living longer doesn't necessarily mean living better. The longer we live, the more challenges we will face physiologically, and the more difficult it will be to live well. Health-care facilities, drugs, and medical procedures cannot help us live better. Only we can.

Death is inevitable, but aging is optional.

Aging is a concept borne out of the human mind. It is not a truth. We can help ourselves live better when we're old.

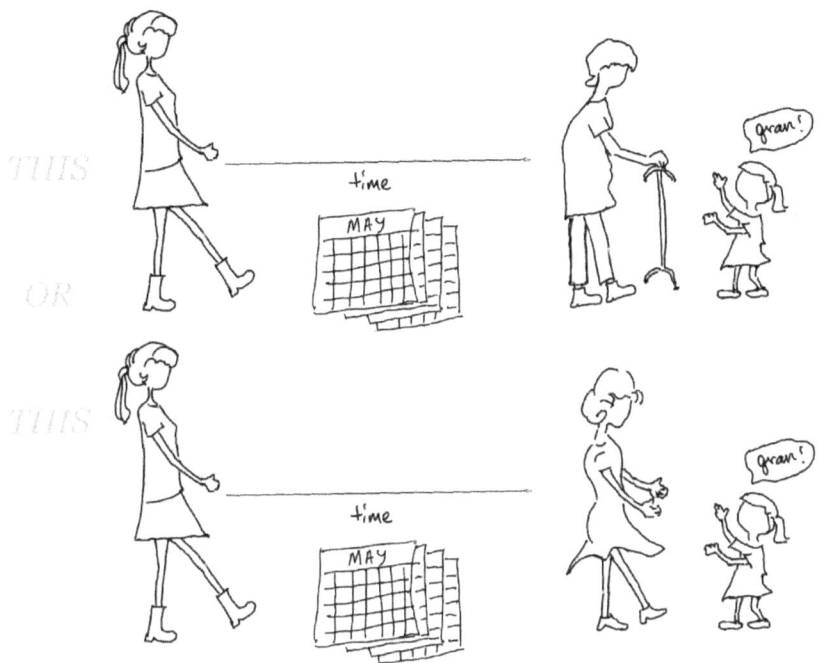

Vicarious Experience

Vicarious experience is the process of learning by observing the experience of others without being directly involved in that experience. For example, we can watch a horror movie. A horrible villain stalks the lady character in the movie. She is scared for her life. Our hearts pound with hers. Adrenaline flows into our blood. We experience her fears. We feel fear even though we aren't subject to any real danger ourselves. In this way, a vicarious experience influences our emotions.

Vicarious experience is a subconscious activity. It affects us physically without our putting any thought into the process.

We experience it almost every waking hour of our lives. Vicarious examples are powerful tools used to influence society as a whole. Companies, organizations, and politicians use it in their marketing campaigns to buy us over.

Sources of Vicarious Examples

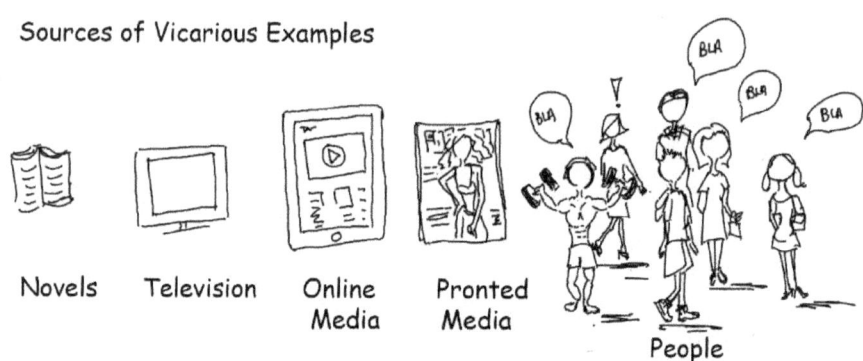

Novels   Television   Online   Pronted   People
                        Media   Media

We learn to age through vicarious experience—by watching how other people age, what other people say about aging, how society in general looks at the aging process. The subconscious mind does a job of it by recording all these external messages of aging. We unknowingly internalize these messages until they become our physical reality.

You can help yourself. Be observant. Identify messages that refer to the aging process—in particular, those that dictate how life should be when a person reaches a certain age.

You can overcome the negative influence of vicarious examples through simple awareness that it exists.

Is there anything positive about vicarious examples? Yes. There are people in our society and in the media who are great examples we can strive to emulate. We can learn something from everyone. With an open mind, we can also find gems of wisdom in others while dismissing the rest of the package.

The Internet is a great resource of inspiring people who know how to keep a young and fit lifestyle. You will often stumble upon them through interest groups and sites dedicated to health and fitness.

Program Yourself to Never Get Old

Getting old is unnecessary and a waste of life. Understand that the concept of aging isn't real; it's an invention of our society. This awareness alone is a leap toward being forever young, forever fit. You can start by reprogramming your mind to change your attitudes about getting old.

Here are two exercises you can do to help you reprogram your attitude toward aging.

1. Make your own lists of what you observe in real life, things that show the differences between an old person and a young person. These may include differences in speech, attitudes toward life, attitudes toward learning, how they plan things, what they do, how they walk, and so forth. Tell yourself you're going to be that person in the young person's list. Those are your attitudes and characteristics.

2. Go to the Internet. Find all the celebrities, sports figures, or people who have certain aspects you admire. It could be their physique, their confidence, their wealth, their charity, or their power. They don't have to be perfect or holy. Paste their pictures on your desktop or create a "vision board" with these pictures.

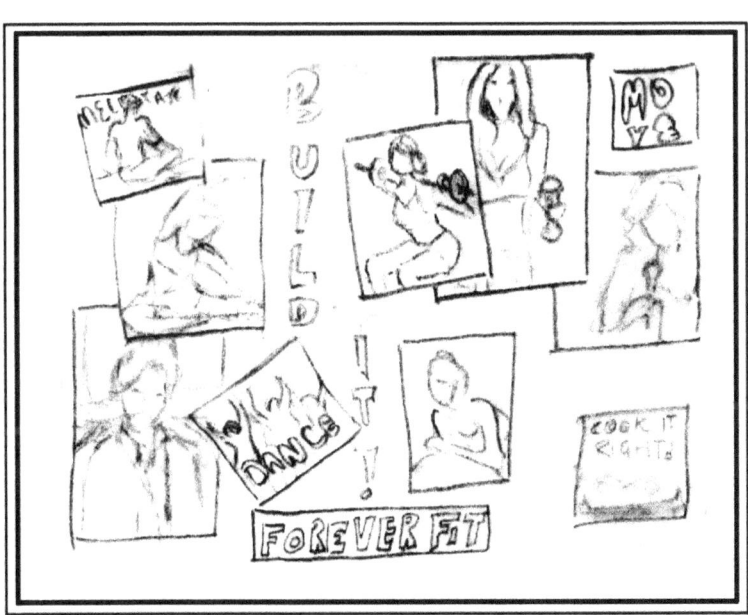

Visualize Your Younger Self

To see in your mind's eye is to believe. Sight is not confined to the eyes. Eyes are merely receptors of light. Photons, which are particles of light, are received by the retina, which sends the data from the light source to the brain. It is in our minds where photons get processed. The brain makes sense of these signals. What we see is really nothing more than our brain's interpretation of the light source. This vision of what we see can sometimes mislead, like the magician's use of optical illusions. The human brain is so analytical that we can read images coming from virtual objects; tiny dots of light from an LED screen become a movie, and splashes of paint become an emotive work of art.

What we really see is not reality but a vision from our mind's eye.

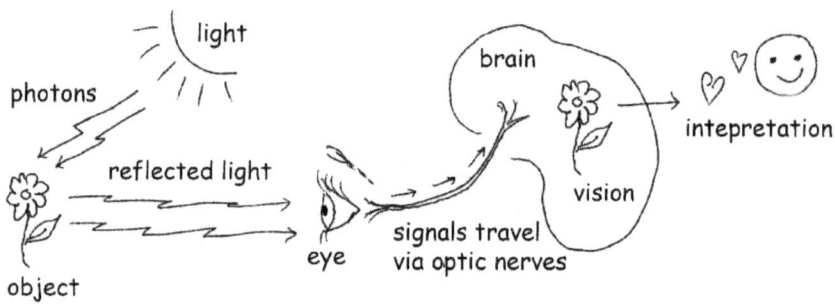

This is how we see things (our vision).

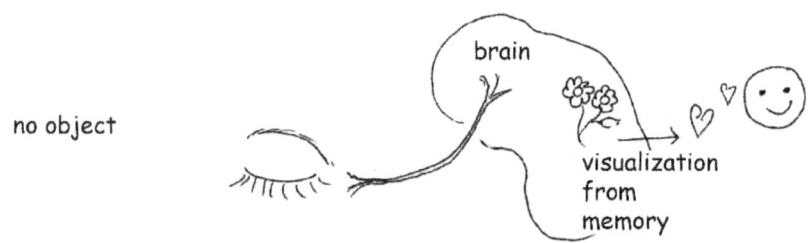

We can also see things with eyes shut (visualization).

When we close our eyes, we can still visualize anything we want. Light is not an essential factor in providing us with vision. Sometimes we call this our imagination. Sometimes it is vivid dreams. Sometimes pictures just pop into our heads, and we call them memories.

You have an expectation. You want to achieve something. You have a goal—a younger, fitter you so you can lead life to its fullest for as long as you possibly can. That goal is a destination. To get to that place, you'll need to have an idea of what that place looks like.

That "place" comes in the form of a younger, fitter version of you. Chances are, you cannot see that you in the mirror—not just yet—but you *can* visualize your potential self in your mind's eye.

The ability to visualize the end point is an important part of achieving goals. This is especially true for goals related to health, for it is the mind that influences the body.

Visualize this transformed version of yourself with this simple meditation exercise.

Before you go into relaxation, create a picture in your mind of what you want to be like after finishing this book. Your dreams are free. Be brave. Dream the biggest most audacious dream. Make this vision of your future self as big as your imagination can take you. Visualize the best you could ever want for yourself.

Got it? Let's start.

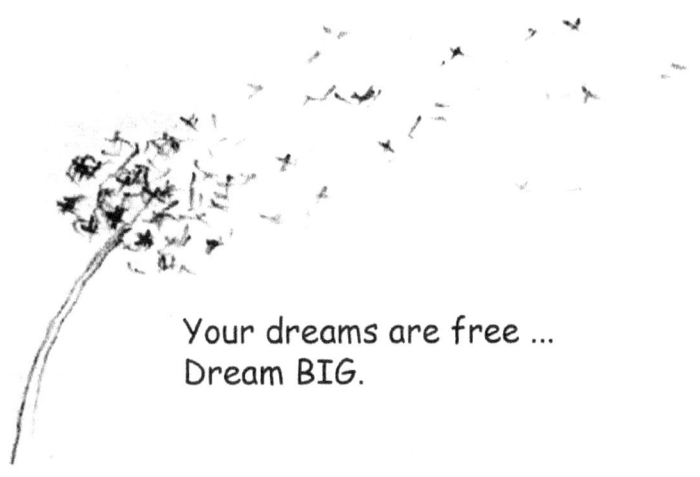

Your dreams are free ...
Dream BIG.

Meditation Technique to Visualize Goals

Sit or lie down in a comfortable place, relax, close your eyes, and let your mind drift. Breathe deeply and slowly. Focus on the breathing until you feel your entire body relax. Think of nothing but each breath you take. Count each breath backward from fifty.

Visualize yourself looking in the mirror. You have changed your lifestyle, and you see that transformed you. The person in the mirror is you. That person is lean, fit, and strong. That is a youthful, happy, healthy individual. Looking at that you, you feel proud with what you have achieved; you have created a great image of transformation. Take more time to admire your image in the mirror. Smooth skin; lean, good posture; relaxed shoulders...and that person is smiling back at you. Take a moment to feel what it is like to be in this strong, youthful body.

Feel the air around that body—feel the skin, the strong muscles, the strong bones, the straight back, that positive energy within.

Maybe this will remind you of a time in your life decades ago, or maybe not. Whatever it is, that is your future.

Feel that new physique, the taut muscles, the straight posture, the confidence.

Hear the oohs and aahs! that come your way.

See your friends be amazed at your transformation.

Hold the sensations.

Breathe. Relax until it is time to awake to your new reality.

Wake.

The more often you visualize, the faster and more effective your results will be. Take your time. Relax. You're on your way to being forever young, forever fit.

You're Already One Step Closer to Achieving Your Goals

You have seen your younger, fitter self in your mind's eye. This vision might be crystal clear, or it might be a little foggy. Whichever way it looks, congratulations—you're really one step closer to reaching your goals. All you need to do is meditate regularly for that vision to get clearer. Practice does make perfect.

This book shares a couple of meditation exercises. They are there because meditation is a great way to de-stress—in this case, to allow your creative mind to visualize and feel your destination. Once you can see where you're going, you can get there without feeling lost.

The Road-Map to that Younger You

To get to that destination, you need to have a special map. Getting young and fit is like going for a lifelong hike. You don't just walk on and on and on, because doing that will just leave you exhausted and burned out before you even reach the halfway mark. You will need to stop at stations along the way, take a break, and congratulate yourself for having made it that far.

Make this book your map. The stations are points from which you can set little goals for you to achieve. You might find some of these chapters easier to take than others. This will be a different experience for every reader.

It doesn't matter how uncomfortable the road will get, as long as you keep moving toward your goal.

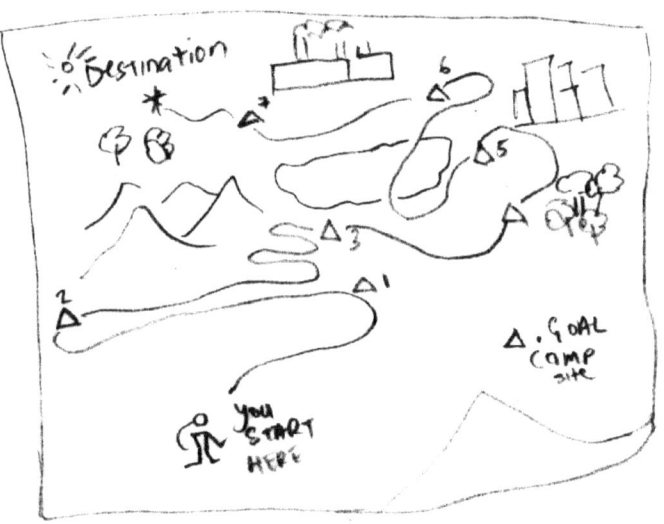

CONVENTIONAL MAP

The Multidirectional Road-Map

The road to getting forever young, forever fit is somewhat different from a conventional map one would take on a hike. When you go on a hike, you move from point *A* to *B*, to *C*, and to *D*—and so on till you reach the end point. Your route is unidirectional, and there is an end point.

Unlike taking a hike, the forever-young, forever-fit journey is multidirectional. In other words, to get to your forever-young, forever-fit goal, you may have to move backward, forward, and sideways. If one goal is difficult to master, keep at it while moving on to the next goal.

Forever is a word that has no final end point. You will keep on achieving goals, set bigger goals, achieve more, look better, get stronger, get more admiration, get more successful, have more energy, and influence more people.

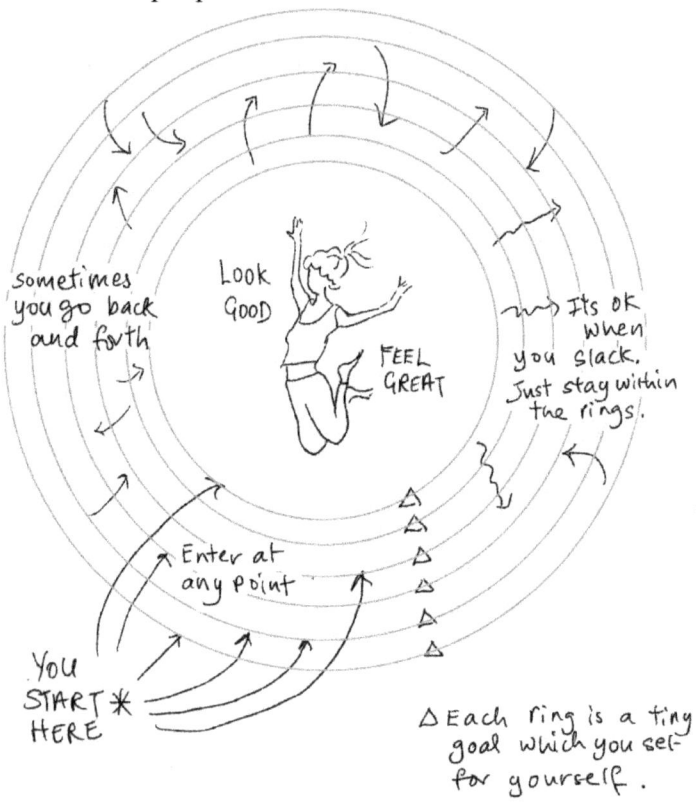

sometimes you go back and forth

Look GOOD

FEEL GREAT

Its ok when you slack. Just stay within the rings.

Enter at any point

You START * HERE

△ Each ring is a tiny goal which you set for yourself.

The FYFF ROAD MAP

Set Your Own Goals

What this book will do for you is highlight the lifestyle changes you will need to make to get forever young, forever fit. It is not a workbook with a timetable of goals set out for you. It is the forever-ness of this project that makes it impossible to create programs that are relevant to everybody at every time.

We're all unique in our strengths, abilities, and motivations. We also have a starting point that is unique to us.

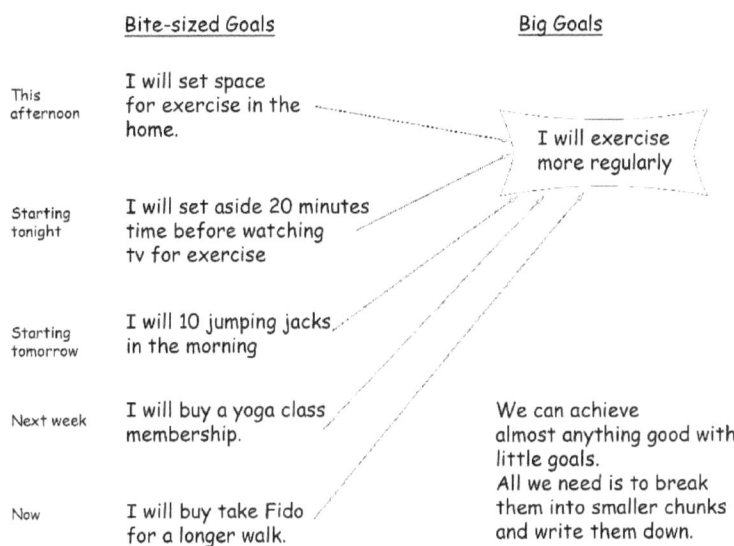

You're encouraged in this book to learn how to set your own goals. Write your own map. Access your success, set new goals, and write a new map. This goes on.

Effective goal setting includes the following:

- Break your project into small, achievable goals rather than trying to achieve everything at once. Small achievements are achievements too. Overcoming small, bite-sized goals can bring as big a success as taking huge leaps.
- Make your goals specific and doable. Instead of saying, "I will exercise more," turn it into, "I will exercise every Friday and Monday at 4:00 p.m." The more specific your target, the more likely you will be at hitting it.
- Remember to always congratulate yourself after having achieved your goals, no matter how small. After all, it is your mind and body making all the effort. At each stage you need to tell yourself that you have done well.
- Forget missteps. If you have fallen back on your goals, gotten lazy, abandoned the journey at some point, don't berate yourself. Slap your wrist and promptly forget it. Pick yourself up and get back on the journey whenever you're ready.

Your ultimate goal is to be able to keep making and achieving tiny goals. Over the years you would have accomplished an enormous collection of goals.

Being able to set your own goals and achieve them fosters independence, leading to eventual success.

"I don't believe in pessimism. If something doesn't come up the way you want, forge ahead. If you think it is going to rain, it will." Clint Eastwood

Don't Stop Believing

This is how your brain works. The human mind is made up of two essential parts:
- The conscious mind and
- The subconscious mind.

The conscious mind is the one trying to do logical things. It gets messages from this book and tries to tell you to visualize your younger, fitter self and set goals.

The subconscious mind is like the little man at the back of your head, giving you all kinds of reasons why it makes no sense to see yourself younger and fitter with age.

You cannot blame your subconscious mind too much. It is responsible for your creativity, gut feelings, intuition, and sense of awareness. It records all your life experiences into your brain like a hard drive in your PC. You need it for survival. It helps you learn from experience and the vicarious examples mentioned earlier.

The subconscious mind doesn't analyze, filter, or differentiate. Hence, not everything your subconscious mind records—such as negative feelings, phobias, and self-doubts—is useful.

If you have thoughts of not being able to achieve your goal of getting young and fit, these are just self-doubts arising from years of environmental conditioning. They come from hearing people say that once you're old you cannot turn back the clock, from watching your parents and friends get old, from observing social and media depictions of old people and aging, from experiencing your own attempts at changing your lifestyle (and ending in perceived failure), and so forth. Be aware that these are just external influences at work.

No past failure is good reason for not succeeding in the future.

The instant a doubt crosses your mind, close your eyes and meditate. Continue reading this book. Work on setting your goals. Believe in the process and the goals you have set for yourself. Believe in your own motivation. That motivation will get much stronger when you start to see positive changes in the mirror.

Believe you can do it, even if nobody is there to go the journey with you. When you start to look younger and fitter, *you* will become the shining example to others. You will become the positive, vicarious example of a forever-youthful-and-fit individual society so badly needs today.

Chapter 2: Time is Not on Your Side

Everything changes, be it material, conceptual, real, or virtual. It is through change that we feel the passage of time. Everything that happens in our lives reminds us of this: the changing seasons; children growing into adults; friends getting old; changes in society, environment, mentality, and culture.

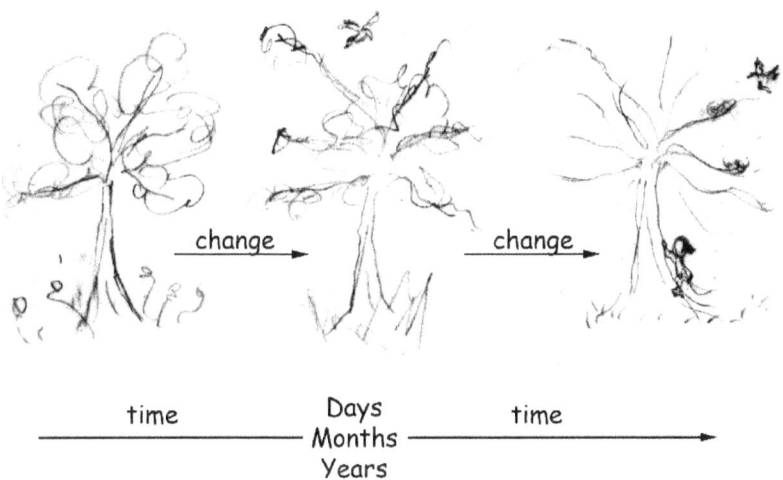

Change moves forward, never stopping, never slowing down. Change is intangible. We invent the concept of time to measure change. Time is not real, but change is.

Aging is the result of a series of changes that take place within the human body. Our bodies are in constant change. It is this change that we address in the pages of this book.

The flow of change is like a massive body of water falling off a high cliff. The energy is so powerful that it cannot be stemmed. We're too weak against this flow of change.

Change is necessary for life to happen. An object that changes negligibly is, in effect, dead.

We can, however, influence the path by which change in our own bodies takes place.

Instead of falling in the direction of deterioration, we have the power to push the change in our bodies toward rejuvenation, regeneration, and development.

Change in our physiology will happen. With effort, that change will be more positive than negative.

Energy and Order

Let's talk about energy a little further. There are two forms of energy:

1. Potential Energy

Potential energy is energy stored within matter. It is also called "latent energy." In this universe, this stored energy is quite unstable. Like the example of the edge of a waterfall, it is like a ball before it falls off a height or a balloon before it pops. Potential energy is the energy required for particles to be held together in an ordered state.

2. Kinetic Energy

When energy is dissipated, the particles spread apart, putting the object into a disordered state. This energy in motion is called "kinetic energy." Kinetic energy is formed when the water falls off the cliff, the ball falls off down from a height, or a balloon pops.

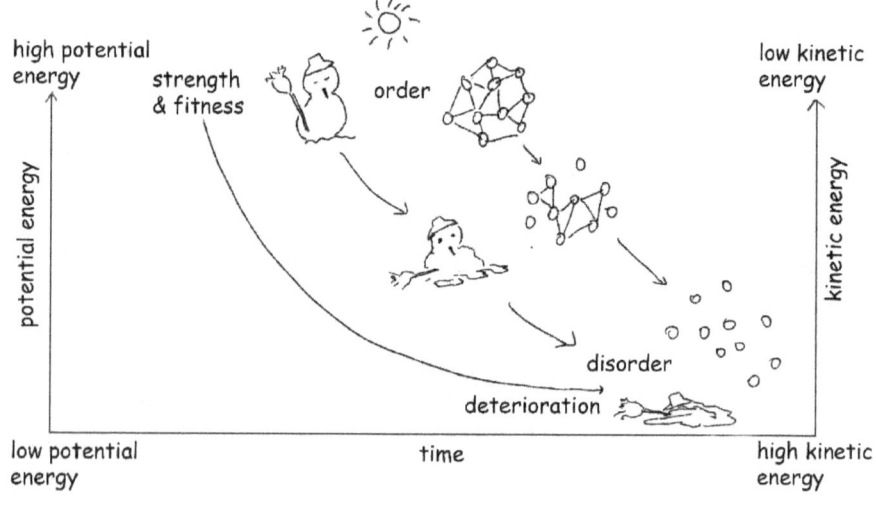

An ordered state is like a snowman. A group of children form the snowman. This act of building a snowman adds potential energy to the figure. The heat of the sun quickly dissipates the potential energy that holds Mr. Frosty in shape.

We see through the melting process that the energy used to hold the snowman together (potential energy) is lost and converted to kinetic energy.

"Letting ourselves go" and getting "over the hill" are the precise metaphors that describe someone who is getting old by implying loss of potential energy—that is, order turning to disorder.

Staying young and fit and looking good are like maintaining an ordered state. It takes energy to keep even ourselves there. This energy is the effort you will take to make the changes.

The good news is that the more energy you put into it, the more successful you will become, because everything will get easier to do.

Since we get more and more disordered with time, it is better to start making the changes as soon as we possibly can.

Staying Young Requires Effort

Deterioration is dispersion of energy. We can loosely relate this to entropy. Entropy is the tendency for energy to dissipate, disperse, or spread out. It describes the tendency of all things in the universe to go from an ordered state to chaos.

Allowing energy to disperse is like letting air out of a balloon. It happens very quickly and with little effort.

Staying young is like blowing a balloon. It takes a longer time and requires more effort to fill a balloon with air than to pop it, because energy is required to keep the air in.

Getting old is too easy. All you have to do is nothing. Remain ignorant. Time will take care of it.

Doing nothing requires little energy.

That is why the larger part of society is convinced that aging is inevitable.

"Just remember, when you're over the hill, you begin to pick up speed." Charles M. Schultz

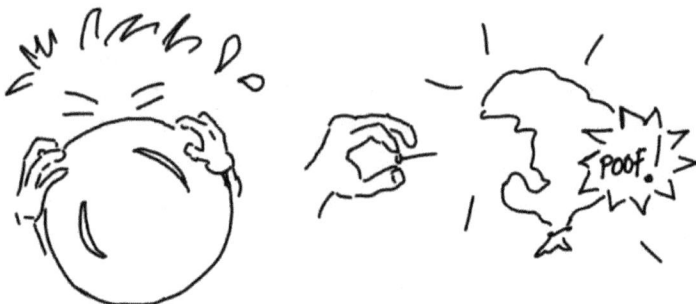

The fact is that looking physically better than the general population does take effort.

We Have the Potential (Energy) to Stay Young

The aging process involves loss of potential energy in your body. This loss of order manifests itself in loss of tissue structure in every organ of the body. That's why people who don't do anything get physically weaker with time.

Doing nothing is a sure way to deteriorate. Putting little bits of time and energy through a lifestyle change will keep you in a more ordered state. This will stem the flow of the aging process.

Effort comes in the form of little goals you set for yourself. These are easy, achievable goals. The best thing is that you will see immediate rewards as you go. You will also find more strength to motivate yourself to go further.

Never Too Old to Start

Today, you're the oldest you have ever been and the youngest you will ever be.

No matter how old you're today, you're never too old to start living forever young, forever fit. You can reverse your own aging process at any point in your life in a natural, holistic way.

The sooner you start thinking *forever young, forever fit*, the easier it will be for you to make the life changes required. The sooner you will get fit, the easier your life will get.

"To exist is to change, to change is to mature, to mature is to go on creating oneself endlessly." Henri Bergson

Not Too Young to Start

You're never too young to start thinking, *forever young, forever fit*. In the previous chapter I mentioned how we learned to get old through vicarious examples. The aging process has already started in your subconscious mind. It already happened at a very early age. You started getting old the moment you were made to understand the concept of aging. It was probably the day you realized Grandpa was old.

A young adult who is unaware of being constantly taught to age is on the way toward the deterioration of the body with time. We don't get old from one day to the next, do we? Somewhere along the way we lose pieces of our youthfulness and turn into old people.

Aging starts with the smallest things, like neglecting our posture, losing muscles, losing interest in new things, looking drab, and getting comfortable with the idea that aging is inevitable.

Then we wonder how we got to become that old person in the mirror.

Even if you think you aren't old yet and haven't a single crease on your face, it isn't too early to start living a forever-young, forever-fit lifestyle.

Understand the urgency. Start now. Begin the process of positive change by understanding the need to put some effort into your new lifestyle. The earlier you start, the easier it will be for you to make changes, and the sooner you will see positive results.

The following chapters in this book discuss what part of your lifestyle needs work. How much work is needed to put the new lifestyle into practice depends on the individual.

You may find that some of the changes are easy to make and accommodate in your life. Some of these habits may already be your second nature. There will also be some changes that will resemble real challenges.

The effort you put into getting yourself forever young, forever fit will pay great dividends. All you have to do is persevere. Time is not on your side. The best time to start doing anything worthwhile is now!

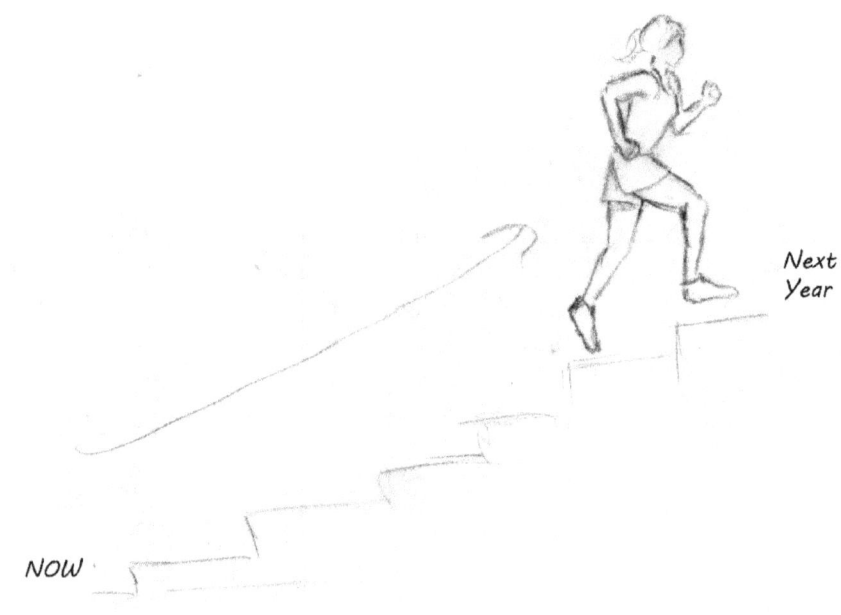

Next
Year

NOW

A year from now, you will wish you had started today.

Chapter 3: Move That Body

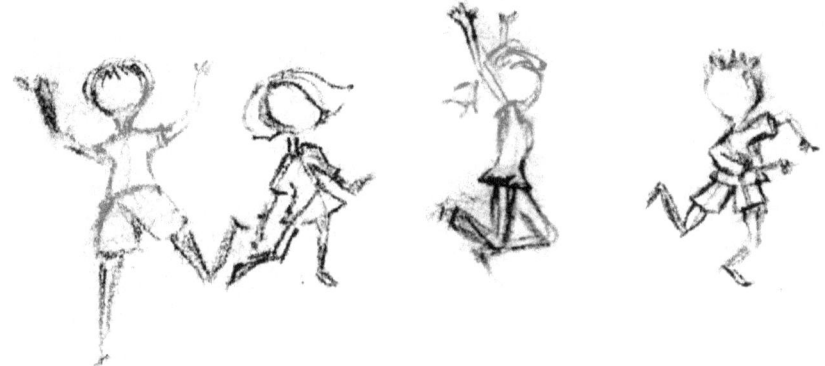

Observe children at a playground. When they are let loose in an environment where they can be free to do whatever they wish, they immediately run off and play with other kids. They will be jumping, running, and climbing for hours if we let them. Kids have no problem moving. In fact, kids love to move around so much that we sometimes have to tell them to be still.

It is an instinct for young children to move their bodies. It is a way we, as young humans, explore the environment. Touching, lifting, and falling are part of the initiation process to life.

As we reach puberty, we become more confident of our physical strength, no longer needing to move like little children to learn about life. In our reproductive years, our instincts shift toward self-actualization.

Self-actualization is our innate desire to realize our full potential. This need to self-actualize really stems from the instinct to reproduce. Just like all living creatures in nature, we try to be our best, look our best, be successful, impress the opposite sex, and intimidate our competitors. Our need for sex drives self-actualization.

Teenagers and young adults move around, often driven by similar goals. For recreation, the guys more likely take part in competitive sports, while the girls engage in more exhibitionistic activities like dance and cheerleading. Young people love to meet in groups, hang out, play sports, go camping, and go dancing, among other activities.

For the majority of people, this level of activity declines, often drastically, when they secure their life partners and the family comes along.

By then, no longer is there time for hanging out in groups; there's no time for sports, no time to dance. We consider ourselves too busy with work, home, kids, and paying the bills.

We call this phase "settling down."

When we settle down, we automatically reduce our need to self-actualize. We automatically stop engaging in activities as we used to.

Our human instinct is also to settle down, build the nest, nurture the next generation, and lose our younger selves.

Settling down usually means stressing out a lot more and moving less, a whole lot less. Some people may say that they still move when they are busy with work, home, and kids. That kind of movement is different from the sort we make when we're teenagers; it is a lot less exhaustive, less enjoyable, more stress inducing, and of little benefit. That is partly the reason why parents tend to gain weight immediately after having children.

Years go by. Children grow up. Some people make more money, some not. Retirement comes.

The change seldom happens from one day to the next, but our ability to move gets progressively inhibited.

Then we watch the kids at sports. We watch them dance and do all kinds of things. Many can be heard saying, "I used to do those things when I was young," because they have come to accept that they are not anywhere as fit as they were before.

The passage of time would have them transform into old, inactive people. Many settle further, get content with being spectators, and watch others live the way they used to live. They may not attempt to take part in some physical activities for fear of breaking something. They get even more sedentary and give up moving altogether.

The larger part of society would agree with this older generation to "stay put," "don't exert yourself," and "at your age, you should take it easy."

But the truth is that "taking it easy" leads to further inability to move.

What if during those in-between years these people had not stopped moving like teenagers? What if they had stayed active in sports, dance, and other recreational activities?

Many would not have found the time to get old.

How different would you be from the majority of people in society today if you had just kept going?

It is rare but not uncommon to find individuals who keep the same physical activity till way past middle age. Many celebrities and retired athletes have kept fit for life.

Seek out good examples of famous people or people in your neighborhood who have kept up with sports and activities that keep them fit. Put their pictures in your clipboard, on your desktop, or anywhere that works as a "vision board."

At any age, do take part in recreational activities, especially those that are fun and challenge you physically. Don't fear exertion.

Never allow age to be an excuse for excluding yourself from the fun. If you already feel physically inept, read this chapter and the next. You can improve your physical condition at any age.

Let's Get Moving: The Little Things first

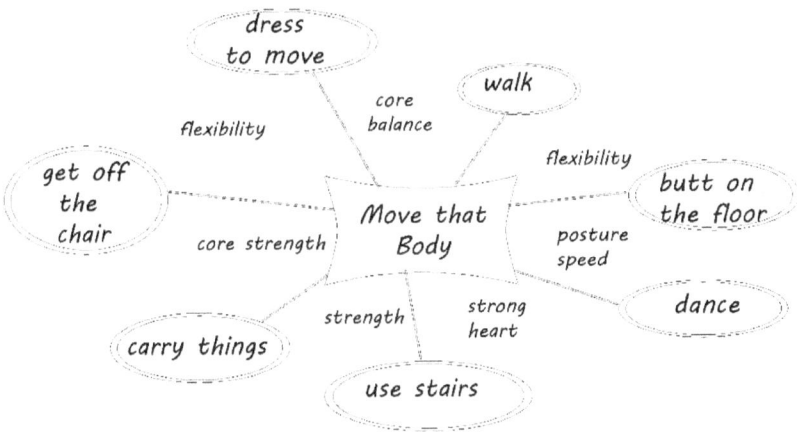

You will probably wonder if I am going to address exercise and workouts at this point. The answer is no, at least not in this chapter. Exercise is really important to get forever young, forever fit, but before that, there is something even more important to consider.

We're going to think about how we move when we're *not* working out. We're going to be conscious of how we move our bodies every waking hour—that is, sixteen hours every day.

Small changes we make during these sixteen hours in a day can make a significant difference in our physical state.

In the beginning, these small changes will seem like effort.

These are small efforts that will become habits if you keep at it.

These habits will be part of your forever lifestyle.

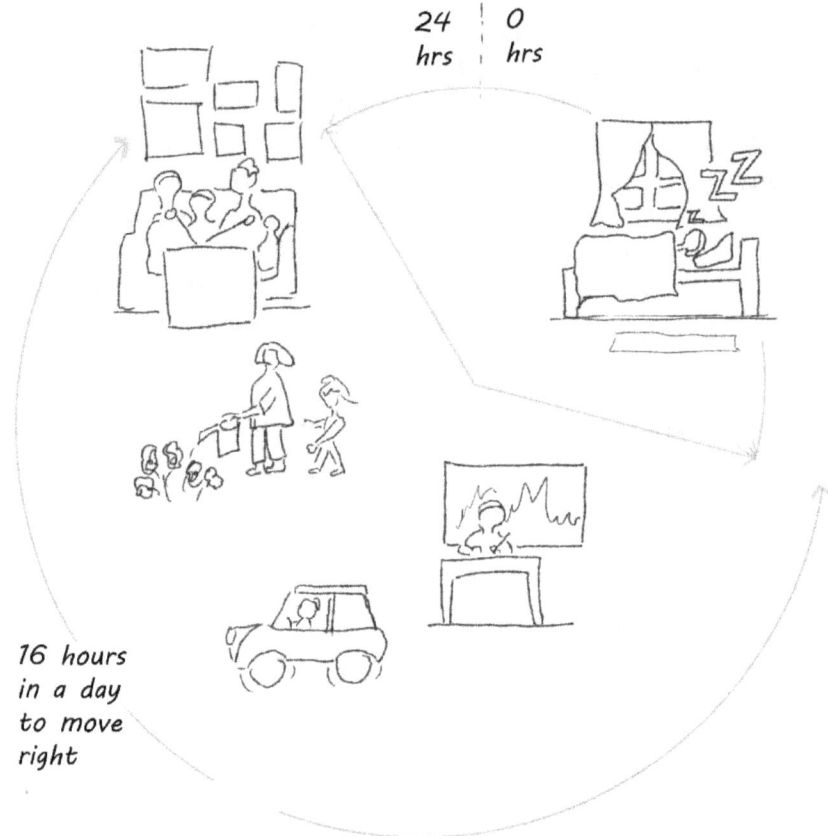

What can these changes do to get you forever young, forever fit?

- Improve your posture.
- Strengthen the core muscles of your body.
- Increase your speed.
- Increase your strength.
- Improve your flexibility.
- Strengthen your heart.

These effects will inevitably lead you toward looking better, feeling more confident, and even being more energetic. You don't need to do tremendous workouts to start seeing changes in your body. You can and should start with the little things. Make these tiny changes as you get on with the sixteen hours of your day.

Dress to Move

If you want to move more effectively, you need to dress to move. Make sure your clothes don't restrict you from movements that involve bending, stretching, and walking.

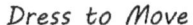

Dress to Move

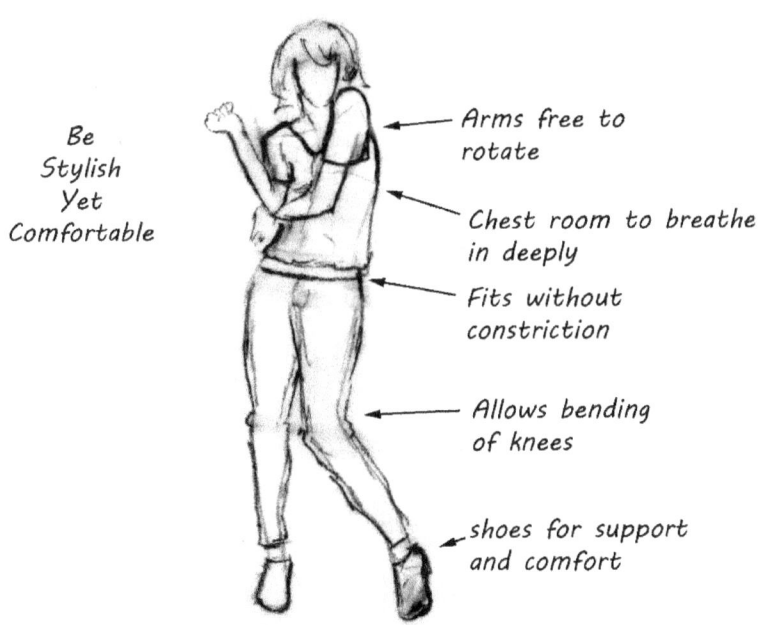

Be
Stylish
Yet
Comfortable

Arms free to rotate

Chest room to breathe in deeply

Fits without constriction

Allows bending of knees

shoes for support and comfort

Clothes that can restrict movement may be the following:
- Pants or skirt that is too tight at the waist or hips
- Shirts and jackets that keep the arms from rotating
- Dresses that are too long and slim, restricting the legs from taking bigger strides (these are typically worn at celebrity red-carpet events).
- Clothes that are so flimsy they make you feel embarrassed to bend over when you need to pick up something
- Uncomfortable shoes

This doesn't mean one should start dressing sloppy and spend days in tracksuits or baggy pants. No. Do still dress to look smart and young (this will be addressed in a later chapter). Clothes should allow the wearer to move right.

Of all the different kinds of clothes that restrict movement, shoes top the list. High-heeled shoes, in particular, are the worst impediments to movement.

"Shoepidity"

I used to feel compelled to wear heels whenever I went out or went to work. I felt annoyed, hampered, and even insecure when I had to wear very high heels. For one, I couldn't walk very fast or very far, or stand for very long in them. Before the evening was over, I was cursing at those "stupid shoes" for hurting so much.

It's crazy to think that we must put up with the pain because society demands it.

After all, everyone wears it. Women who wear heels tend to have an air of feeling superior to others. We even think we look better when we look at ourselves in the mirror with inches-high stilettos on; the higher the heels, the nicer the image appears on the mirror.

The problem is, when we look at ourselves standing in front of the mirror, we're not walking.

The higher the heels, the more awkward the walk. Awkward walk is ugly. There is nothing more pathetic than a woman trying so hard to look good and only undermining that look by walking like an invalid on stilts.

When we walk on high heels, the balls of the feet are forced to absorb all the body's weight. This absorption of body weight on a small set of bones on the balls of the feet adds pressure to the knee, hip, and spine. This pressure, in turn, causes the core muscles in the body to compensate as we walk. Over time, as our core muscles (muscles in the torso) are forced to balance our body in this unnatural way, our postures will be altered. It will be altered from a natural state to an unnatural state. This unnatural state will ultimately lead to pain and injury.

Long-term high-heel-shoe wearers often complain that they can no longer walk on bare feet. That is a sign that the tendons and muscles in the calves and ankles have stiffened up, rendering the feet inflexible. This inflexibility can affect your ability to balance. That will lead to ungainly gait and falls.

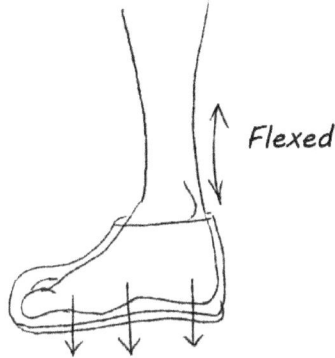

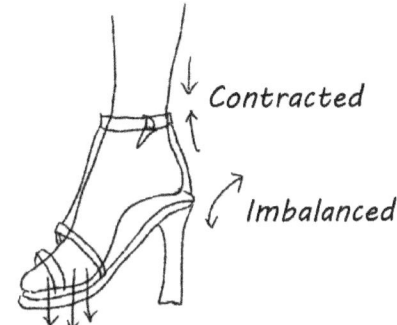

Flat soled shoes –
the pressure on the
foot is spread out

High heeled shoes–
the pressure on the
food is concentrated
on ball of foot

Walking is a vital human movement. If the muscles required for walking are impaired, staying mobile is very difficult for us. We need to wear sensible shoes that allow us to walk like healthy human beings. These need not necessarily be ugly sneakers. Many great brands of shoes are beautiful yet sensible.

Sensible shoes allow you to do the following:
- Walk with the right posture.
- Walk briskly.
- Keep your balance on uneven ground.
- Avoid slipping.
- Walk a distance.

Someone who is young and fit walks right, with footsteps and posture and gait to reflect vitality and health.

Walk This Way

Walking in the right way is a sign of youth. Anyone can spot a young, strong, and fit individual from a distance just by the way he or she walks.

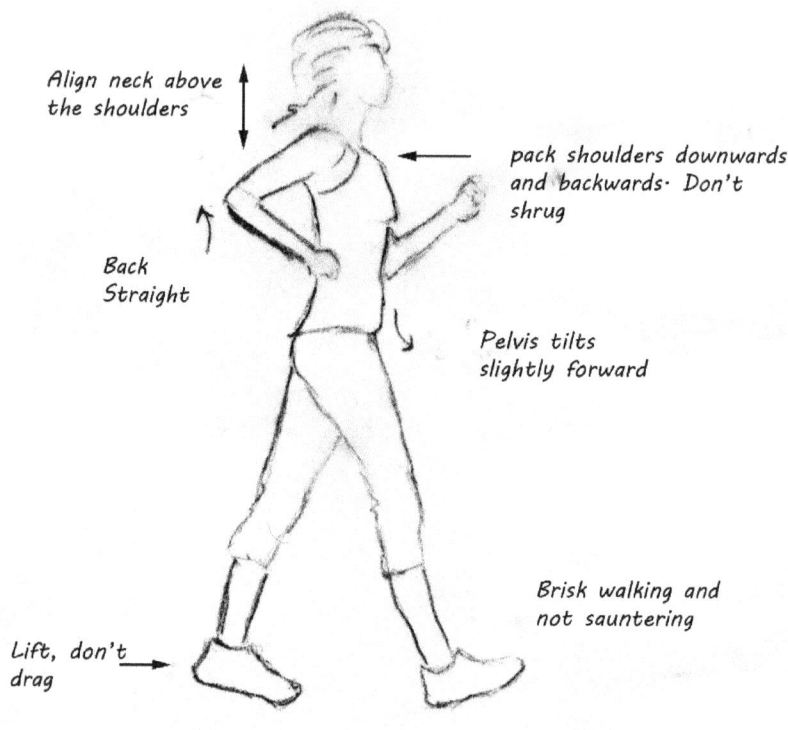

Align neck above the shoulders

pack shoulders downwards and backwards. Don't shrug

Back Straight

Pelvis tilts slightly forward

Brisk walking and not sauntering

Lift, don't drag

Here are some rules to remember when walking:

- Align your neck above your shoulders. Don't move the head forward or backward turkey-like.
- Pack your shoulders by first pulling them backward and downward. Squeeze the blades together. You will see your chest rise a little.
- Engage your core muscles (the muscles that hold up the chest, back, sides, and stomach). Pull your stomach muscles inward, pressing your belly button into your body toward your spine.
- Tilt the pelvis forward. Think of Michael Jackson's famous dance move—pushing his pelvis forward and back. Push your pelvis forward and keep it there. When you walk, your butt should not be sticking out.
- Walk as briskly as you can. Sauntering and feet dragging are nasty habits that can make us look old, weak, and lazy. Walking briskly

ensures that we stay energetic at all time.

In the beginning you may find walking like this to be a bit strange. That is because muscles in the body had been taught to work the wrong way. Keep practicing your new walking posture and pace. Take long walks walking like this. Soon walking right will become a habit.

When you're mindful of how you walk, you will not only get from place to place faster, but your cardiovascular strength will improve. The muscles in your legs, back, and abs will strengthen. You will look young and get fitter just by walking properly.

Get Off Your Chair

We have become chair shaped. The chair is the most ubiquitous furniture in our homes and work environments. Can you think of a typical day in your life without sitting on, or being in the presence of, a chair? If you can, you're probably living in the wild or in a backward rural community. You may also have the advantage of better posture than the rest of us.

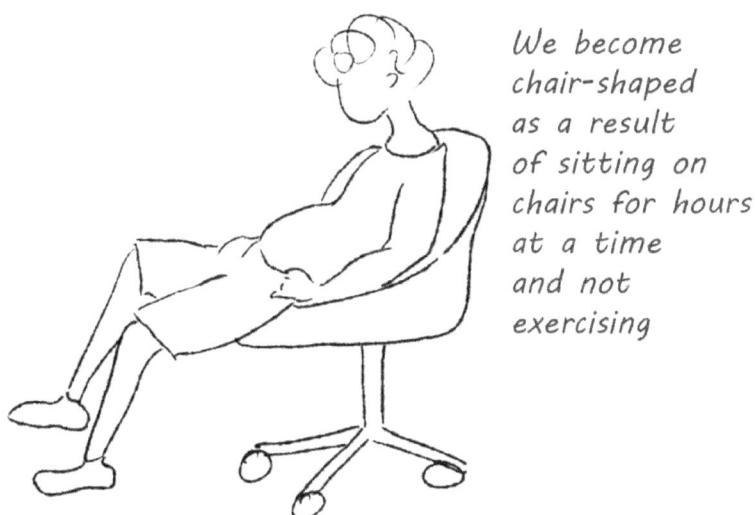

We become chair-shaped as a result of sitting on chairs for hours at a time and not exercising

The chair is a human invention. Most of us spend hours each day sitting on some kind of chair. The fact is, human beings by nature are supposed to sit on the floor, sit on a piece of rock or a log, or squat. Sitting on chairs for long stretches of time makes us chair shaped.

Usually we end up slouching forward or backward. The spine isn't held in its natural s-shaped curve.

There are two main problems associated with being chair shaped:

- Muscle weakness. This causes muscle imbalances in the abs and back (the core muscles). Some muscles will weaken because of lack of use. The weak muscles will lose their ability to support our spines. That will prevent us from having the right posture. Poor posture robs us of mobility; doing simple things like walking will be difficult and ungainly. Poor posture is dangerous because it can trigger back injuries just by the way we bend down and lift objects.

- Inflexibility. Being chair shaped renders the muscles along the back and legs inflexible if we don't have the habit of sitting on the floor or squatting.

Reduce the length of time spent sitting. This will prevent your posture from deteriorating any further. Instead of sitting on the couch while watching television, try sitting on the floor. Better still, do some stretching exercises while you're at it.

In the office, sit on a stool instead of a soft chair. Every couple of minutes, go take a walk, climb some stairs, or do some jumping jacks or push-ups.

Sitting less on chairs is a small step toward your goal.

Get (Your Butt) On the Floor

People from Asia are in general more flexible than people from the West. People in rural Asia sit on the floor a lot, like you see in old-fashioned Japanese and Korean teahouses. In schools kids in Asia still sit on the floor for some lessons. People there also (till recently in most cities) use squatting toilets. That is why Asians are by nature more flexible than people in the West.

Sitting on the floor is the natural way for human beings to sit. We overuse chairs so much so that we no longer have the flexibility to get on and off the floor. If sitting on the floor is a difficult position for you to get into, you have lost your innate ability to move right. It is time to get off the chair.

Flexibility is important for mobility and balance. You need to be flexible enough to sit on the floor comfortably. This will help you move more effectively, get up from falls, and even break falls in the first place.

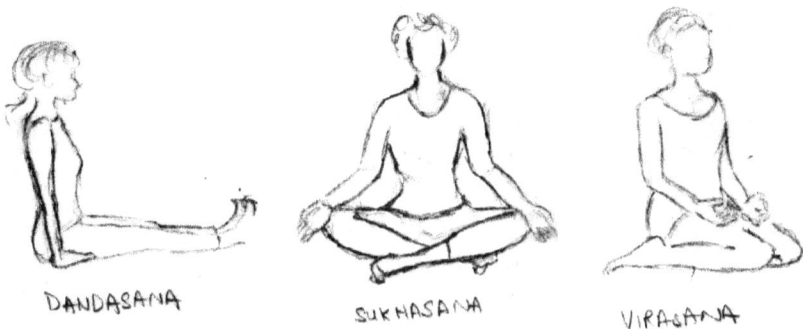

DANDASANA   SUKHASANA   VIRASANA

You also need to be able to get into a squatting position. This is the natural position by which human beings used to do their private business. Modern-day people, of course, use toilet seats and hence don't need to squat in the toilet.

This doesn't mean we can go through life without being able to squat. The squatting position takes us from and off the floor. If we're too rigid to squat, we will have problems with mobility and be susceptible to falls as we age.

The best way to be able to squat is to practice it every day, little by little. Use a sturdy support (like a wall, a sturdy chair, or a railing) to hold in front of you while you get into a squat.

There is no need to overstrain. Just practice a little every day.

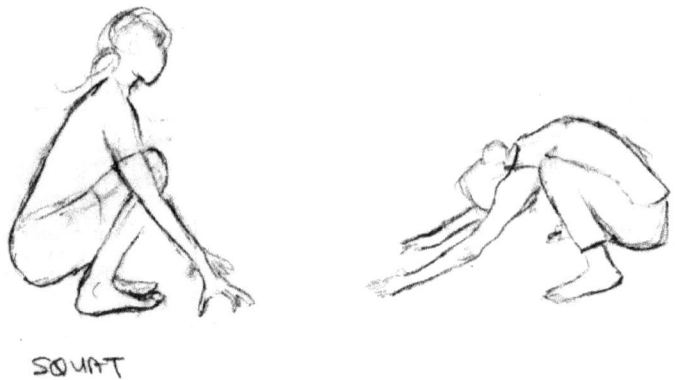

SQUAT

These could be the most important mobility exercises you will need for your legs and back. Being able to squat and sit on the floor will help you to do the following:

- Gain muscle strength in your legs and back.
- Gain balance, which prevents falls. The effect of falling can be reduced if you're flexible enough to bend your limbs and absorb impact.
- Gain flexibility and hence more mobility. You get a wider range of motion when your muscles are supple. Being able to bend and stretch allows you to break falls.

Use the Stairs

If you want a quick fix to getting fit, losing lots of fat in a short time, use the stairs. Stair-climbing is the most-exhaustive, low-impact activity you can do with your legs. It even makes for a multilevel workout on its own. It develops strength in your legs and core muscles. Those big thigh muscles hold up your skeletal structure. The cardiovascular benefits are considerable even at a low pace.

Make using stairs a habit whenever the opportunity arises. How much of a workout you want to make of it will depend on how fast you climb or how many flights you take.

Whatever it is, use it. It will get you places. You're young and fit if you remain able to walk up flights without too much difficulty.

Carry Your Own Bags

Lifting is a necessary movement. We need to carry things to get through the day—from our groceries to our kids and things we need to move around.

It is important to remember the previous pages in this chapter about movement, posture, and strength. Those are important points if we want to be able to do these tasks of lifting safely.

While in the next chapters we will cover lifting exercises, we can address lifting as a habit.

Just like using stairs, carry your own bags. Don't avoid the activity by getting others to do it for you or by using trolleys for every small thing you should be lifting instead.

Consider lifting a privilege and lift more. It will strengthen the muscles in your upper body. Just remember some important points:

- Avoid lifting anything that is too bulky or heavy.
- Keep your back straight when lifting even the smallest thing. Tighten the muscles in your abdomen. You can help keep the spine straight by tilting your head up and fixing your gaze ahead of you rather than on the floor. Your hips, spine and neck should be in alignment. Inhale deeply before lifting the weight, exhale as you lift.
- Keep your knees soft and slightly bent as you lift heavier objects off the floor. Engage your thigh muscles as you lift.

If you have flexibility problems, work to improve flexibility by doing squats and stretches before lifting anything. If you feel that you cannot tighten the muscles in the abdomen or thighs, it shows that your muscles are weak due to lack of use. If you feel your spine sag in the middle, don't lift anything. Rather, move on to the next chapter on exercise.

If you're moderately healthy you can strengthen your shoulders, upper back, and arms every day by carrying your own things.

Dance

"Rhythm is the basis of life, not steady forward progress. The forces of creation, destruction and preservation have a whirling, dynamic interaction." The Kabbalah

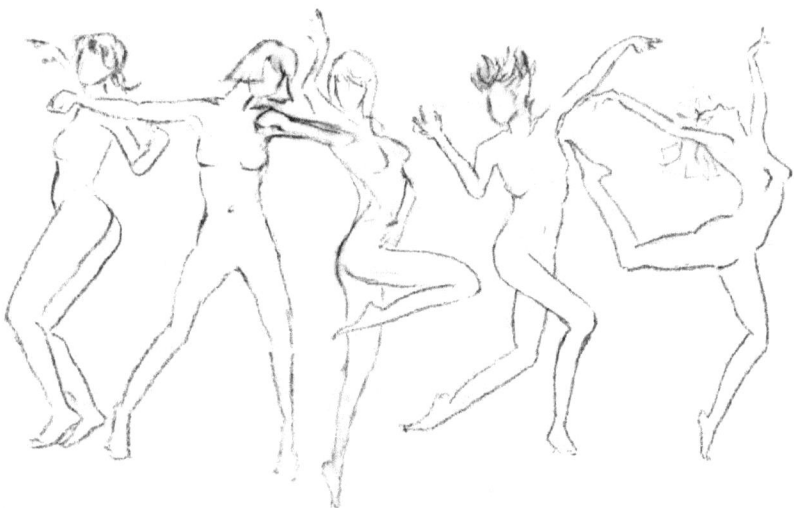

Dancing is a natural human instinct. Humans have been moving their bodies to a beat long before we invented music. We possibly invented rhythm through dance.

We're no different from our early ancestors, who used dance to get themselves into a state of trance. *Why would they do that?* You may ask. They got into trance for a variety of reasons, from recreation to experiencing spirituality and healing. Being in a state of trance is no different from complete relaxation; the kind of pleasurable effect we get in deep meditation. Getting into trance naturally has many benefits like rejuvenation of the body, and the opening up of the mind. In today's world we can get into an extreme state of trance through a destructive practice taking addictive drugs. Unlike natural trance, trance under the influence of narcotics doesn't bring benefits because they break down the body's natural ability to rejuvenate itself.

As we dance our minds switch focus from the mental state of constant thought to moving the body to the rhythm. Depending on how deep we're "into the groove," we actually get into a state of trance. We may not feel anything strange or different while dancing, but we may feel a slight sense of enjoyment, and pleasure. Sometimes we get so into it that we forget time. That is a trance experience.

While dancing alone with soothing music can be relaxing, dancing with loud music and together with a crowd gives us a heightened experience. In a dance hall with strobe lights, the thumping of bass, the beats of the music, actually puts the crowd in a collective state of trance.

Being in a trance state sets the body in a flow. When our bodies are able to move freely to a beat, we release our physical inhibitions. Freedom of the body leads to freedom of the mind.

We will discuss the importance of de-stressing in keeping young, fit, and ailment free.

Anyone can dance. Each of us has his or her own natural way of movement.

You get the best of your dance by freeing your mind while focusing on the beat of the music. When the body moves, the mind stills.

When dancing at home, wear comfortable clothes. Go barefoot. Start with stillness, then move like you're flowing. Enjoy the dance.

Remember in dance always to respect the body's boundaries. Dancing for relaxation is therapeutic. It is relaxation through movement. It is not meant as strenuous exercise.

With dance, you achieve stress relief, mobility, and enjoyment. When dancing with others, you also get good company and a heightened state of trance.

Use It to Keep It

The mind controls the human body. The mind is powerful. The mind decides to do things. The mind can decide to move the body. When the mind keeps telling the body to move, the body decides that its muscles, bones, organs, and tissues have purpose.

A sedentary lifestyle is a signal to the body that not all is necessary. In this state the body conserves its energy and stops renewal processes. It starts to "settle down."

When you're in this state, you lose your muscles, cardiovascular strength, and suppleness. Your bones also thin out. On the surface you will look like an old person.

The opposite would happen with constant movement: the mind sends messages to the skeletal muscles to build more muscles, blood keeps pumping, tendons stay supple, cardiac strength increases, and bones stay dense. You're in effect staving off degenerative diseases like osteoporosis and heart disease.

The less you move, the less you will move. It is a vicious cycle. Limitations in mobility has very little to do with age but with lifestyle.

Never relinquish your right to move.

Society tells us that slowing down is a consequence to getting older. We can choose to believe that, or we can open our eyes and look around for good examples of individuals who just keep going.

Under normal circumstances, a person who keeps physically active will never lose his or her mobility from one birthday to the next.

Even if things change for the worse—say, for example, the person gets sick and has to spend months in recuperation—he or she is still better off dealing with the physical trauma than being like an individual who leads a sedentary life. He or she is also better able to get back into action once his or her state of health returns to normal.

Staying mobile is a strategy for survival. Our prehistoric ancestors had no choice but to keep moving or starve and get eaten. All we need to do in today's world is to keep moving to live better.

Why then do people in general slow down and die?

This could be the result of unconsciously giving up on progress.

How often do we hear of a woman or man who was just divorced or widowed and suddenly seems younger because she or he "is back in the game"? This is an example of how a change in relationship or marital status can lead to change in mind-set, from "middle aged with grown-up kids" to "a single person looking for mate." People in this situation suddenly start to dress better, hang out more often with other young people, play sports, go dancing, exercise more, and so forth.

I am reminded of the Kevin Spacey's character, Lester Burnham, in the movie *American Beauty*. Having fallen for his daughter's teenage friend, he transforms himself into somewhat of a middle-aged hunk.

We certainly don't need to go through life-changing experiences to start moving. The opposite actually holds true.

When we take more interest in life and get physically active, the good life will find us.

Awareness of the need to keep our bodies in motion—taking part in sports, fitness, exercise, and dance—is a big step in staying young and fit. We can all make conscious efforts to use as much of our physical power to be healthy and active every day of our lives.

Chapter 4: A Stronger Version of Yourself

It is a universal understanding that being physically fit is paramount to staying young and feeling great. The only way to achieve this goal is through regular exercise. This chapter will encourage you to exercise regularly in an efficient way and with the right spirit.

Fitness—What Does It Mean?

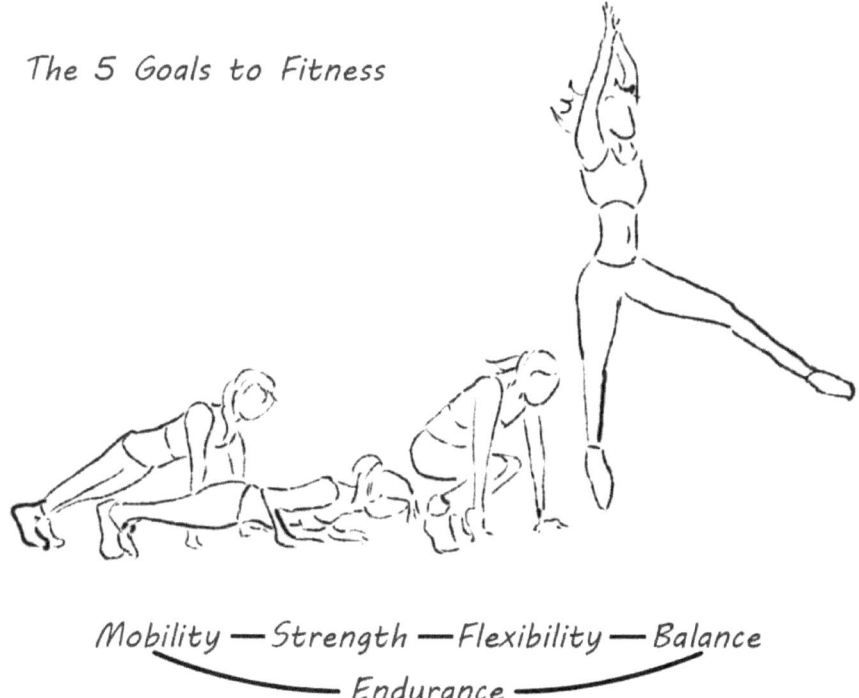

The 5 Goals to Fitness

Mobility — Strength — Flexibility — Balance — Endurance

Fitness is a state of health that involves attaining the following physical attributes:
1. Strength—The power in your muscles to do work like lifting, pulling, pushing, and holding on to a position
2. Mobility—The ability to move your body from one position to another. This property encompasses strength and flexibility as well as the element of speed.

3. Flexibility—The ability of muscles and connective tissues to stretch. Flexibility is an essential factor for mobility and the prevention of injuries.
4. Balance—The brain-to-muscle coordination that allows us to hold our position without falling
5. Endurance—The measure of cardiovascular fitness. It is important to gain endurance so you can engage in physical activities without getting too easily exhausted.

Endurance is what most people quite wrongly consider to be "fitness." It is an important element in fitness, certainly, but it is only useful together with strength, mobility, flexibility, and balance. These fitness attributes are best developed and maintained with regular, mindful exercise.

Your Road to Fitness

The purpose of this chapter is to provide you with an understanding of the real purpose of physical exercise. Since we all start at different levels of physical fitness, you will not find textbook prescriptions of which exercise you should do, when to do them, or how long your exercises should take. You will be provided with enough information to plan your own workout and training routines as you develop physically.

Fitness is not about getting thin.

Your Body is Unique

The body is in constant dynamic change. Every individual is unique. Your body will develop on its own terms and respond to exercise in its own way. How it develops varies at different times in your life.

Enjoy your uniqueness. Don't make the mistake of comparing your development with someone else's. Some people grow muscles more quickly than others; some need more cardio to get lean. Others just stay thin and wiry. Contrary to what some exercise gurus might like to have you believe, there is no exercise routine in the world that would work for, or bring the same results to, everyone every time.

You're embarking on a lifelong journey. There is no end point.

There is no thirty-day, sixty-day, or ninety-day magic. Exercise programs that use a time frame make only marketing sense and work mainly to encourage us to exercise consistently for the time period. That is the "pro" of these programs.

The "con" of this is, after that what are you supposed to do?

Having a personal trainer is probably the best way to get started in exercise. If you can afford the expense, it is well worth the money. A good personal trainer will educate you on the right type of moves and the exercises you need to match your present physical condition. He or she can also be a great motivator to keep you on your exercise program.

Not everybody can afford the luxury of having professional help. That is perfectly fine as long as you understand there is such a thing as doing the right kind of exercise and that you need to keep motivated. In the following pages, you will get an idea of how exercise to get fit works. You will also learn how to do it and how to get yourself motivated.

For most of us who are not in the habit of exercising, this is the chapter of greatest challenge. This is also the chapter offering the highest reward.

Start with an open mind. Rethink everything you've been taught about exercise and read on.

Regular exercise is a good way to reduce excess fat, but getting thin is not the point of exercise; rather it is to be young and fit. It is a false belief that thin people are healthier than fat people.

Regardless of our body shape, the majority of us need to set time aside for exercise.

Why We Need Exercise

The Environment
The environment we live in today doesn't engage us adequately to stay fit. We sit in chairs for hours each day. Our muscles don't stretch enough to stay flexible. We don't get to lift anything heavy enough to stimulate the muscles and bones to regenerate and grow. We don't walk on unstable surfaces long enough to regenerate our nerve fibers. Neither do we run, climb, or jump to strengthen our cardiac muscles.

Longer Life Expectancy
Medical science has made it possible for us to live longer. This advancement poses a challenge for us to live healthy and independently into our nineties. We need exercise to build the physical resources so we can live better as we get older.

Obesity
Our environment is making us fat. Food and lifestyle cause us to store up more energy than ever. Needless to say, fat accumulation is a cause for concern because it leads to chronic illnesses and a poorer quality of life. We need exercise to expend this excess energy.

Stress
Exercise relieves stress. Pumping of blood into muscles stimulates the flow of hormones that, in simple terms, inhibit stress-hormone production. Many of us don't even realize we're living under stress. Stress is dangerous, as we will discuss in later chapters.

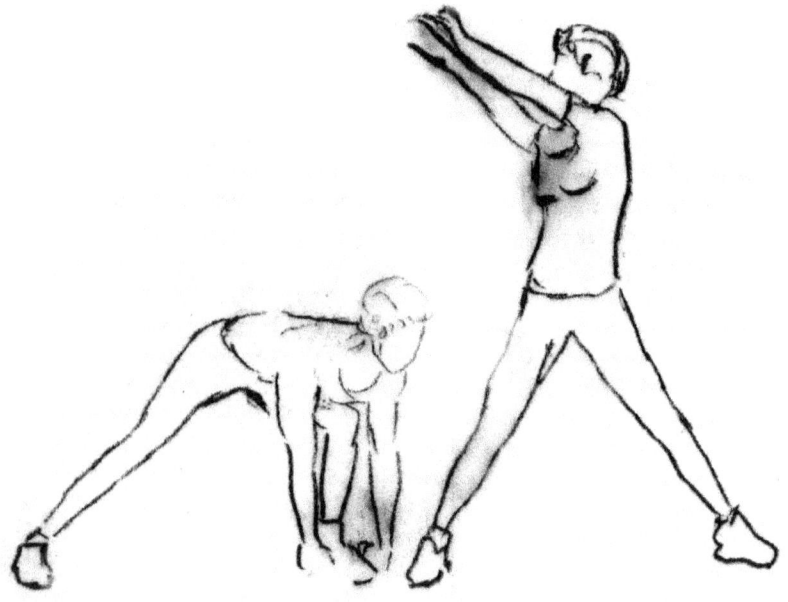

How Exercise Really Works in Anti-Aging

Aging is a process of loss whereby attributes of strength, mobility, flexibility, balance, and endurance deteriorate. For most people this deterioration begins in their early twenties. It is perhaps true that the human body has evolved to gradually lose its level of fitness with age.

This phenomenon is due to the decreased secretion of growth hormones in the body over time. The pituitary gland produces growth hormones. Factors such as age, gender, diet, stress, sleep, and exercise affect the amount of hormones produced in the body.

The good news is that by having the right diet, sleep, stress management, and regular exercise, we can naturally stimulate the production of growth hormones in our own bodies.

The Function of Growth Hormones

Research has shown that the functions of growth hormones include the following:

- The stimulation of muscle growth
- The increase of bone density
- Lipolysis (the breakdown of fat in fat cells)
- Protein synthesis (for the building of tissues—for example, skin, ligaments, and so forth)
- The stimulation of the immune system
- The decrease of the liver's uptake of glucose and the increase of glucose production for energy
- Homeostasis (balance of body fluid condition in the body);

Growth hormones are responsible for building and replenishing cells and tissues. In humans, these hormones are necessary for growth until we reach reproductive age. When growth is no longer the priority, the body conserves energy by producing fewer and fewer growth hormones.

Lowered growth-hormone production results in reduced ability of the body to rebuild and replenish itself. The results are visible signs of aging.

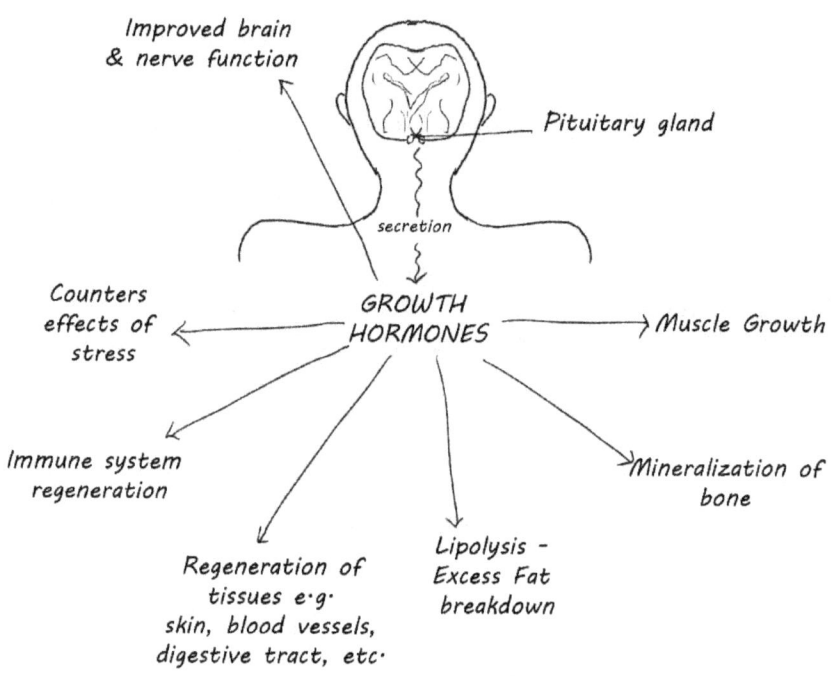

Production and function of growth hormones.

It might seem like we're programmed to gradually shut down. Since we know the physiological effects of growth hormones, we can do something about this problem.

You can stimulate your body to secrete vital growth hormones naturally.

Studies have shown that we can increase our body's natural production of growth hormones through the following activities:

- Participating in regular strength-building exercise
- Controlling blood sugar by cutting refined carbohydrates and sugars from the diet
- Getting adequate amounts of relaxation and deep sleep

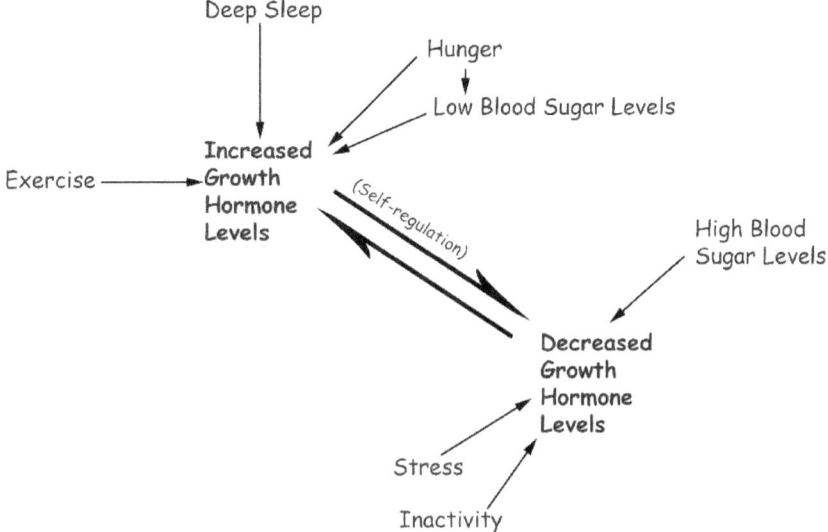

This is the reason why people who exercise regularly have an easygoing personality, live a relaxed lifestyle, and tend to look younger than their peers. These people live lifestyles that naturally boost growth hormone levels in their bodies.

The reason for exercise is to cause a rise in human growth hormone levels.

Hormones are chemicals produced in specialized cells in the body. Their function is to transmit messages to their target cells so necessary biological functions can take place. Each hormone is produced in cycles, like the ebb and flow of the waves in the ocean. The human body produces a variety of hormones. These hormones work synergistically to enhance or inhibit the effects and secretion of each other.

Growth hormones are affected by the presence of other hormones. If growth hormones are necessary for maintaining good physical form, then we should try to maintain healthy levels of these hormones.

With the passage of time, lifestyle habits affect the hormonal profile in the body. Knowing the key hormones—their regulation and effects—will guide us toward making healthy choices.

Exercise, Workouts and Training

There is a difference among exercise, workouts, and training.
An *exercise* is a movement you perform. For example, you may do some jumping jacks. That is an exercise.
A *workout* is a series of exercises you may do in succession and in one sitting.
Training is a program of workouts that are planned for a term.

Reps, Sets and Intervals

Reps—or repetition—in exercise is the number of times an exercise is repeated continuously.
A *set* includes a number of reps of the same exercise. This is usually followed by a short period of rest and then another set of the same or different exercise.
An *interval* is the amount of time required to complete a set. It is usually measured in seconds.

Frequency, Duration and Intensity

When planning a workout routine, there are several factors to consider:

Frequency is how often someone works out each week.
Duration is the measure of how long each workout session lasts.
Intensity is how hard someone work. This is normally measured by one's heart rate during exercise and the feeling of exertion.

Get into the best shape of your life. Aim to work out three to four days each week. Make exercising a routine. It will become a habit once you get into the groove of it, and the benefits will become apparent. All you need to do is stick to a plan you set for yourself.

Frequent workouts with few rest days keep your metabolism at a moderately high level, thus enabling the body to naturally burn excess calories. Working out four out of seven days each week may seem like a lot, but the most effective workouts take forty or less minutes to complete. That means less than a total of three hours per week for workout time. That isn't really very much considering how much time most of us spend on the couch, watching television or surfing the Internet.

Intensity and Duration

Intense, short workouts of twenty to forty minutes per session done three to four times each week are more effective than one three-hour workout done once a week.

The Importance of Rest Days

Rest days are as important as exercise days. During rest the body regenerates itself, builds muscle mass, cleans away toxins, and burns excess fat. You need your rest days, especially if your workouts are intense. On these days it is especially important to have a clean diet (which we will discuss in chapter 5), lots of water, and sufficient sleep.

Listen to your body. Rest when you need to rest.

The Weekend Warrior's Pitfall

"Weekend warriors" do nothing physical all week and then decide to run three-hour marathons on the weekends. This routine fails as it does not help build fitness or health. Here's why:

- A three-hour workout done once a week is ineffective in building true physical fitness. If one lasts three hours at a stretch, the person is really not pushing hard enough. Workouts become most effective when the intensity level of the exercise allows no more than a few seconds of continuous movement at a time.
- On and off physical activity often leads to injury. Long periods of lack of exercise tend to leave muscles dormant. Sudden strain on those muscles can lead to injury.
- Long-drawn-out exercises tend to be repetitive. An example of such an exercise is jogging, which involves using the same set of muscles repeatedly with the body weight constantly pounding on the same joints. Instead of building, the exercise

is actually wearing out parts of tendon, ligaments, and cartilage.

- Extended workouts drain the body of fuel. When the diet is not in check, the body burns protein together with fat. While burning fat is the aim of the weekend warrior's exercise, the protein depletion eventually becomes his or her undoing. Burning protein depletes muscle and other essential organs, leading to degeneration and aging. Since muscles are the powerhouse of energy burning, losing muscle foils efforts to stay lean.

- You're more likely to miss out on your workout if you allot all your workout time to one session. It is like putting all your eggs into one basket.

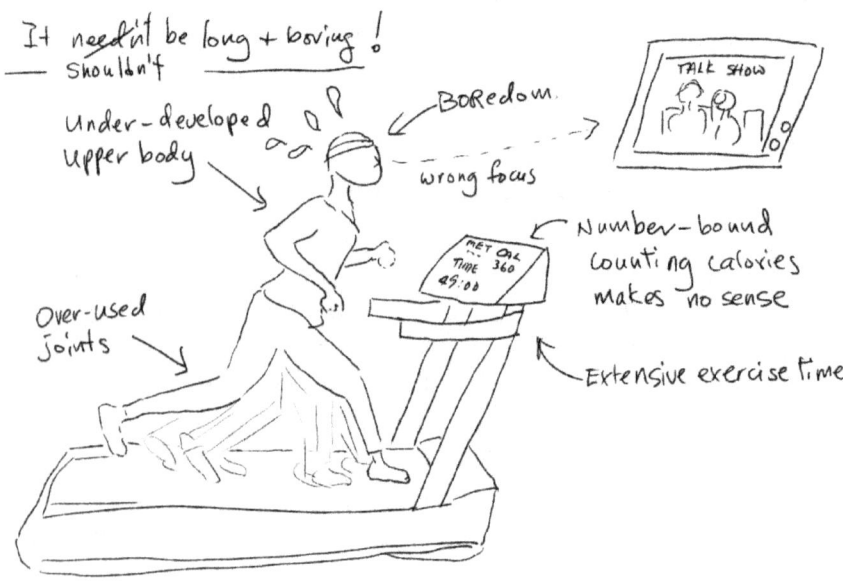

Getting-Started Motivation

There are several ways to get regular exercise into your life. Every person can set aside about thirty minutes, four days a week, for workout by the following:

- Watching forty minutes less of television
- Spending forty fewer minutes on the Internet
- Spending forty fewer minutes chatting
- Hanging out forty fewer minutes in bars, cafés, and shopping centers

Pick one of the above time-wasting habits and decide to dedicate that time to your workout. Make it a routine. Fix that exercise time. Make a plan for the week. Make a workout diary.

The best time of the day to work out is the time of the day you're most likely to work out.

Your Workout Diary

Get yourself a diary just for your workouts. Plotting down a week's workout in advance would help you resist the temptation to do anything ad hoc in place of the session.

After you complete the planned workout, put a check mark beside the date.

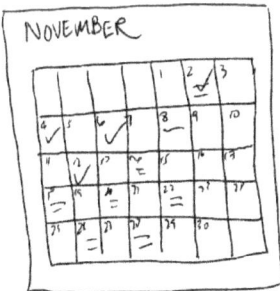

In your calendar, plot out your workout schedule a week in advance. This will help you avoid doing anything else in place of exercise.

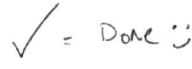

Plan Your Workout

Before your workout, jot down the type of exercises to do for the session as well as the number of sets and reps for each set or interval. Here are some examples of workout plans:

Workout Plan 1	
Jump-rope	50 secs
Rest	10 secs
Squats	50 secs
Rest	10 secs
Burpees	50 secs
Rest	10 secs
Burpees	50 secs
Rest	10 secs
Repeat x 4 Rounds	

Workout Plan 2	
Jumping Jacks	20 reps
Crunches	15 reps
Burpees	10 reps
Squats	20 reps
Plank Hold	for 30secs
Repeat x 3 Rounds	

Workout Plan 3	
Pushups	4 reps
Crunches	4 reps
Burpees	4 reps
Squats	4 reps
Repeat x 20 Rounds	

You can plan your workout any way you like. Get ideas from the books or the internet. Keep it challenging and fun.

Exercising Right

Your exercise should lead you to a life of youthful fitness and health. There is no other real purpose for doing the exercise other than to stimulate growth-hormone production for replenishing organs and tissues.

Good exercise is about getting fit. Truly fit.

You will defy the process of aging by looking good, staying lean, being physically stable and mobile, and staving off illnesses linked to the aging process.

Exercises that build muscle mass will ultimately help you keep the fat off. Increasing muscle mass increases your resting metabolic rate (RMR). This means that the more muscle tissue you have in your body, the more calories you burn off throughout the day, even during the time when you're sedentary or asleep.

We shall go through the different exercise concepts to ensure we understand how these actually work.

Strength Training to Grow Muscles

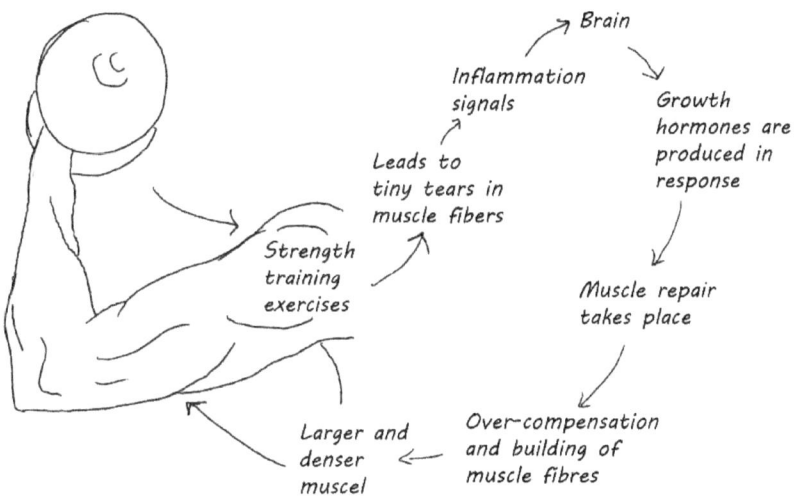

Brain

Inflammation signals

Growth hormones are produced in response

Leads to tiny tears in muscle fibers

Strength training exercises

Muscle repair takes place

Larger and denser muscel

Over-compensation and building of muscle fibres

The Effects of Strength Training

Strength training is for everybody. Numerous studies have shown that people, no matter how old or weak, can start to gain muscle strength through strength training. Strength training is also very effective for building muscle mass.

Strength exercises can be done with or without the use of weights. Exercises without the use of weights or equipment is sometimes referred to as body-weight training. Body-weight exercises are the best exercises to do because they are fuss free; there is no need to go to the gym or have any equipment on hand to do body-weight exercises. All you need is a little space to work out.

There is a variety of equipment available on the market for the avid exerciser. All equipment is useful to those who use it.

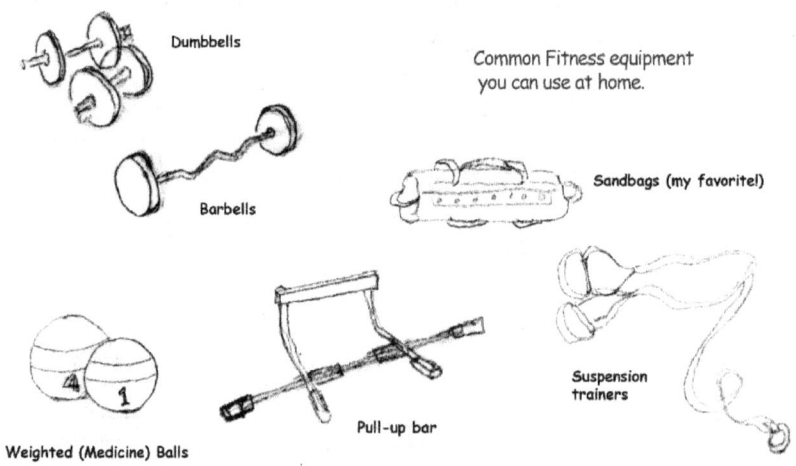

Dumbbells

Barbells

Common Fitness equipment you can use at home.

Sandbags (my favorite!)

Suspension trainers

Weighted (Medicine) Balls

Pull-up bar

Weight-training workout routines have the following characteristics:
- They vary in duration. The focus is on lifting, pulling, and pushing. Hence the time needed to complete the workout is not of the essence.
- They vary in intensity. To be effective, weight training must be intense. Work to your maximum for best results.

You can increase intensity in the following ways:
- Increasing weights
- Increasing resistance
- Doing more repetitions
- Doing exercises more quickly or
- Doing exercises dead slow

Weight-training exercise are useful for everybody because
- they are low-impact exercises suitable for most people;
- they are easy to get into if you're an absolute beginner to exercise;
- they build muscle mass quickly and therefore upgrade your growth-hormone production;
- they are ideal for people with cardiovascular issues; and
- they are great for very thin or fat people.

The following pages present examples of effective strength-training, muscle-building exercises. These are done using free weights or just your body weight.

There is so much you can do—so many interesting moves for your workout. If you're a complete beginner, it would be best to engage a personal trainer. The alternative is to read books dedicated to workouts and exercise or to catch some exercise videos online. There is an updated list of books and links recommended at our website, www.foreveryoungforeverfit.com.

Doing it Right

Strength training is for muscle building. It can come in the form of heavy dumbbell lifting or small controlled movements using your body weight.

Do keep good form at all times. A total beginner at exercise is best advised to engage a trainer or have someone help with the exercise techniques.

Push yourself but don't let ego take over and overstrain. Exercise is effective if there is effort. This effort must be borne out of mindfulness.

Use simple free weights like dumbbells, barbells, sandbags and weighted balls, rather than fancy gym contraptions. These simple equipment neither restrict natural posture nor provide unnecessary support to the body. There is an advantage to this because when free weights are lifted during exercise, the muscles must work hard to keep the body in balance. This extra work will engage entire sets of muscles simultaneously. A balanced musculature is what we want to achieve from our exercise.

Do exercise that include compound movements rather than targeted movement. Compound movements make use of a large group of muscles at a time. This is natural movement. Exercises that use compound movement create balanced musculature. Examples of compound movements include squats, lunges, burpees, lifting free weights, lifting, pulling and pushing heavy objects from one point to another and push or pull-ups. These are actually simple exercises that mimic the kind of movements we engage in daily activity.

Exercise that only "target" individual muscles are best avoided. These exercises include exercise that engages only one set of muscles at a time rather than engaging full sets of muscles simultaneously. Usually these exercises make use of a bench to sit or lie on, and rely on complex gym machines. These are exercises commonly done by body builders for the purpose of building definition in some muscles quickly. The danger of isolating muscles during workout like this is that while some muscles get pumped up, the others remain weak. This state of imbalance often causes injury. When the exerciser needs to make natural movements in lifting, his or her less developed muscles might overstrain and snap. Do try to understand this philosophy of doing compound exercises and use commonsense while exercising. Think. Do the exercises you're doing feel like natural movement, or do they seem to be awkward?

Exercises should be challenging but they have to feel natural. If a movement causes you to feel discomfort, discontinue the exercise. It could be that the movement is not right for your posture, or it could be that your muscles aren't ready yet. There is such a thing as doing simpler exercises first, then slowly progressing to more advanced workouts. It is better to seek help with training, but if help is not available to you, do some research online or with help of reliable exercise books.

Vary your exercise. It is often tempting to keep doing the stuff you're already good at. That doesn't help keep you really fit and may even leave muscles lopsided. Variation is also more fun than doing the same thing over again. I would recommend using the internet as a resource for good ideas. There are many fitness bloggers and free workout videos for those who want more exercise routines.

Keep Your Movements Natural

When doing strength training, always bear in mind to keep your movements natural. The best exercises are those done with movements that feel like a natural flow.

Watch your form. Your back should be straight and your torso muscles tight.

Move deliberately. Don't swing or throw.

Use appropriate weights. You should feel like you're lifting, pulling, holding, or pushing something that is heavy enough for you to do eight to twenty repetitions at a time.

You may find it necessary to seek advice from a professional to get your form right.

The following two pages illustrate a variety of exercises you can do to work the entire body for true fitness.

The images in the following pages show some exercises to get you started. These exercises work to reinforce natural body movement. All these moves have a purpose—to strengthen sets of muscles evenly so you can perform daily tasks such as lifting grocery bags, carrying children, getting up from the floor, or climbing a flight of steps with ease. They are compound movement exercises that engages sets of muscles together rather than a single muscle in isolation. You will develop stability and strength from working your body this way.

Body-weight exercises require only the use of your body; you don't need to be in a gym or spend money on equipment. These are exercises you can do anywhere—outdoors, indoors, and even in a hotel room. These exercises are enough to get you fit.

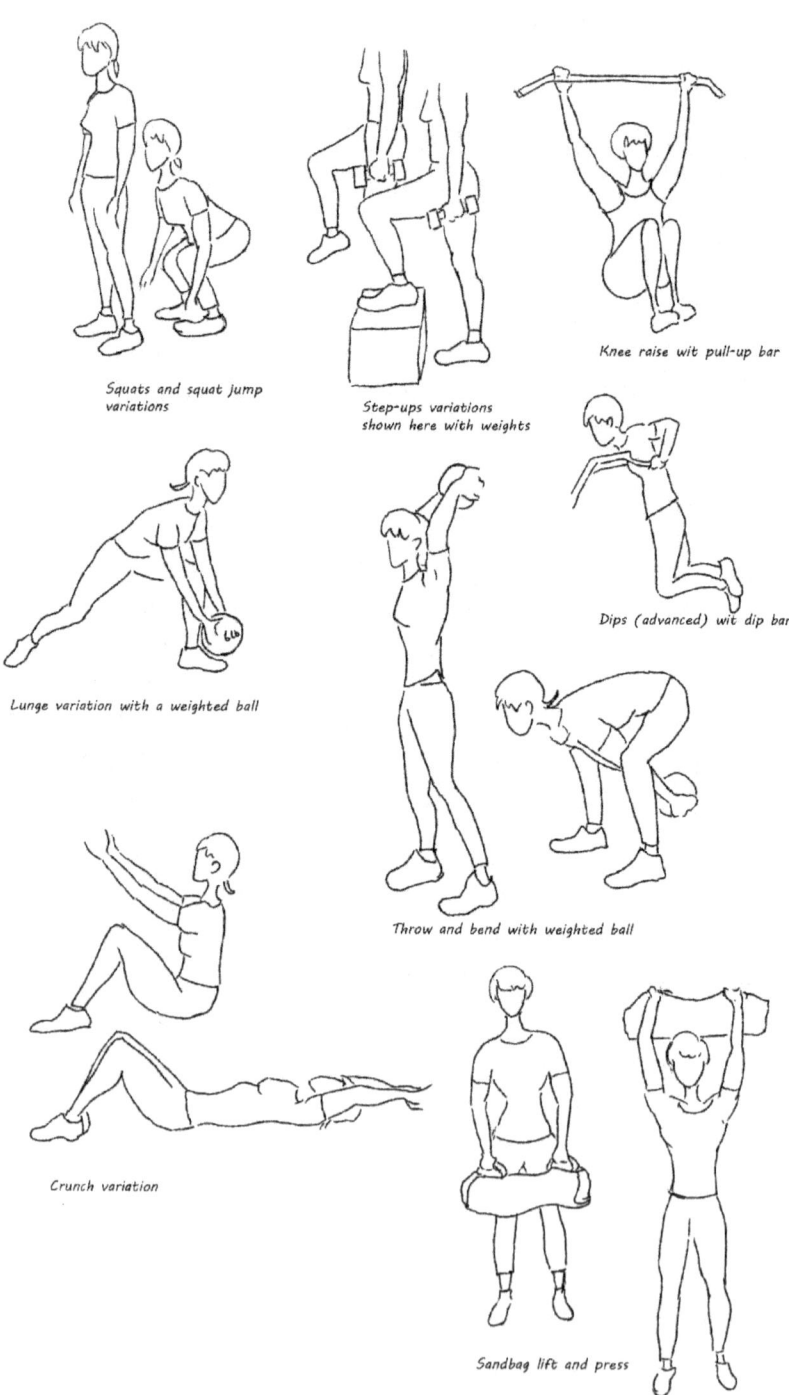

Squats and squat jump variations

Step-ups variations shown here with weights

Knee raise wit pull-up bar

Lunge variation with a weighted ball

Dips (advanced) wit dip bars

Throw and bend with weighted ball

Crunch variation

Sandbag lift and press

Illustrations of the types of exercises we can do with simple or no equipment. Please consult a professional trainer to learn the right forms. The moves should feel natural.

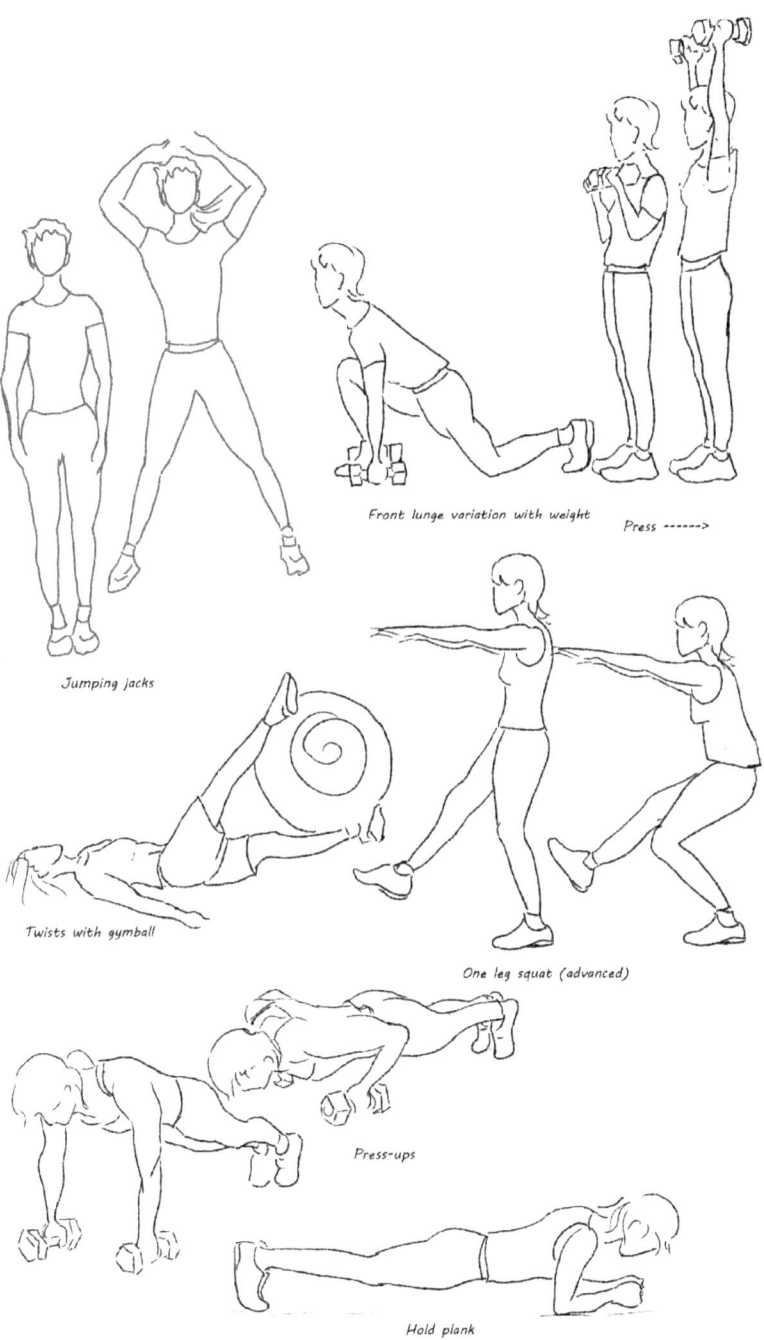

Front lunge variation with weight   Press ------->

Jumping jacks

Twists with gymball

One leg squat (advanced)

Press-ups

Hold plank

Illustrations of the types of exercises we can do with simple or no equipment. Please consult a professional trainer to learn the right forms. The moves should feel natural.

Burpees!

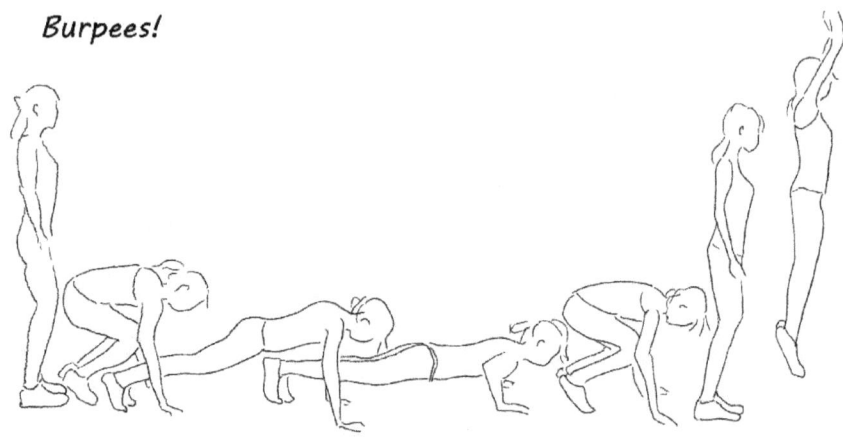

The above exercise move is known to many as a burpee. It is my favorite exercise. This is a great exercise that works the entire body. It strengthens legs, arms, back, and abs. The movement is explosive because you have to repeatedly jump up from the floor and go back down again. This improves cardiovascular endurance. There are also variations we can make with this exercise; for example, we can incorporate push-ups, jump squats, and leg tucks. For beginners, the burpee can be done at a slower pace. For added challenge, we can lift dumbbells and sandbags while doing a burpee. The burpee is ideal for times when you need to warm up or get into a workout mood.

Interval Training for that Cardiovascular Oomph!

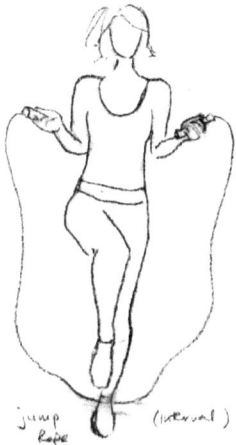

Interval-training sessions include very short-duration, high-intensity workouts. Commonly known as high-intensity interval training, or HIIT, these exercises seem like a cross between strength training and cardio exercises, but the focus is on doing as many reps as possible in a specified time (the interval).

The exercises are done with a timer, which is set at twenty to fifty seconds of "work" and ten to thirty seconds of "rest." During the "work" interval, you should do an exercise as quickly as possible. For example, do as many jumping jacks as possible on the beep of the "work" interval until the timer beeps again to start the "rest" interval. Catch your breath on the "rest" interval. On the next beep, do another set of exercises as fast as possible for the "work" interval. Most HIIT workouts last thirty minutes or less. You can get a good session in with just twelve minutes.

HIIT workouts are meant to be intense, and they are most efficient for fast results toward a lean, strong body. They are, however, not suitable for everybody. Absolute beginners might find HIIT almost impossible to do. If that is your experience, keep up the weight training but at a slower pace. Over time you will gain enough strength to do HIIT.

Interval-training workout routines are characteristically short in duration. The main advantage of short workouts is that they don't encroach on your life. Short workouts are easy to keep doing. Everyone can spare minutes in a day for an activity that is so important for maintaining good health.

HIIT builds cardiovascular strength. To work to one's fullest effort at every interval, speed and effort are of the essence. The heart rate rises during the "work" interval and recovers during the "rest" interval.

HIIT also builds strength and agility. There is more focus on speed and, depending on the exercise, dexterity. Body-weight exercises like burpees are great additions to interval training.

Due to its intensity, and depending on your level of fitness, interval training is optional and can be incorporated into your workout schedule.

Exercises you can do with HIIT include running sprints, running up the stairs or hills, using a jump rope, doing jumping jacks, using a stationary bike, as well as doing burpees, squats, step-ups, push-ups. Almost any kind of body-weight exercise can be incorporated into a HIIT workout.

There are several ways to plan. Here are some examples to help you understand the concept of interval training.

Interval Training

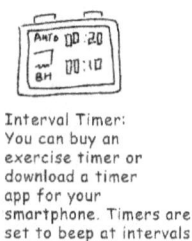

The exercises A, B, C and so forth, can be varied or the same moves.
A good workout would last 12 to 20 minutes in total.
During the short 20s of exercise, work as hard and fast as you possibly can.

Interval Timer:
You can buy an exercise timer or download a timer app for your smartphone. Timers are set to beep at intervals while you exercise.

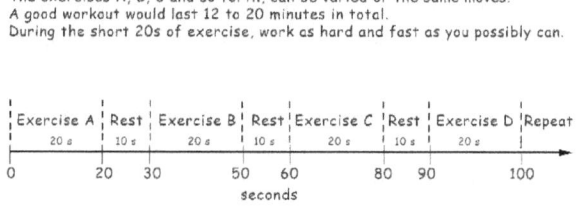

This is an example of a twelve-minute session. You can change the session time or the intervals:

• Set your timer to ping at twenty-second and ten-second intervals. In the twenty seconds, do an exercise as quickly and with as many repetitions as you can. For the next ten seconds, rest.

• On the ping of the next twenty seconds, do the same exercise or another exercise. For the next ten seconds, rest.

• If you do this for eight rounds, your exercise session will last exactly four minutes. If you really worked as hard as you can, that would be four minutes of intense exercise.

- Repeat this process 3 times, and you would have completed a very intense 12 minute HIIT session.

  Here are variations you can make with your workout:

- You may change the intervals—for example, fifty seconds of work and ten seconds of rest or fifty seconds of work and twenty seconds of rest.
- You may do more rounds or fewer rounds (longer or shorter sessions.)
- Change the exercises. Vary the moves.

Interval training is versatile. The only thing to remember is to use your best effort. If you work to the max, your workout session shouldn't exceed forty minutes. Most of us would keep it at less than twenty minutes.

As you get fitter, increase the intensity of the exercise by

- increasing the speed of your moves;
- progressing to more advanced exercises by changing the range of motion or adding weights;
- extending the work interval; or
- shortening the rest interval.

High-intensity interval training has been proved to be the most effective exercise routine to gain strength, mobility, and endurance while burning excess calories in the shortest time.

"If you always put limit on everything you do, physical or anything else, it will spread into your work and into your life. There are no limits, there are only plateaus. And you must not stay there, you must go beyond them." Bruce Lee

Yoga

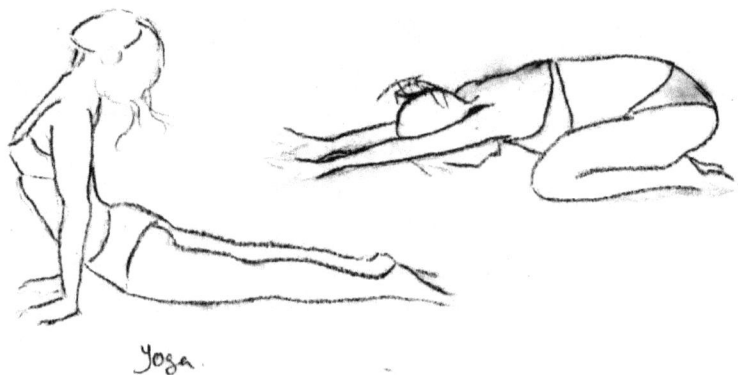

Yoga.

Yoga exercises combine strength, flexibility, balance, and even meditation. There is less focus on pushing and pulling heavy weights or seeking cardiovascular intensity as in strength training. In yoga, the poses are controlled. The muscles are activated by staying in a contracted state while holding a pose. There is a lot of focus on the form of the body. Doing yoga regularly helps flexibility and balance, two very important aspects of fitness.

If there is movement, each repetition is done at a very slow, controlled pace, with attention to breathing. Duration is usually as long as strength training or longer. More advanced yoga sessions can be up to ninety minutes long. The intensity of exercise in yoga is multilevel. It is not common for weights to be used. In such cases, intensity is increased with more advanced poses and/or a longer length of time by which the pose is held. The advantage of yoga-type workouts is that their movements don't put high impact on the joints. Yoga is ideal for healthy individuals as well as those with special physical needs.

Muscle density can be built with isometric exercises. A long duration of muscle contraction encourages the growth of new muscle fibers—which builds strength.

Regular workouts of this kind encourage growth-hormone production, which in turn brings about anti-aging benefits.

Flexibility exercises that come with most yoga programs enhance mobility like no other.

These exercises are not as aerobic in nature as other types of training. Calories are not "burned" as quickly during workouts. However, as with other strength-building exercises, muscle mass is built, thereby raising the RMR, which ultimately results in a leaner physique.

With the right program, muscle mass built over time from these workouts will result in strength, mobility, flexibility, and a leaner body composition.

Yoga should be part of your fitness regime. You can incorporate some yoga moves during your rest days or some stretch-and-balance poses as a cool-down routine after a workout.

Vary Your Workout

The body has the tendency to get used to repetitive workouts. To prevent that "plateau effect" and get best results for your efforts, it is important to make variations and change things around every couple of weeks. Here are some changes you can make to your routine:

- Slow down each move. Strength-training exercise gets difficult when done in a dead-slow pace. Try doing a push-up so slowly that you would take thirty seconds to complete a repetition, and you will realize how difficult it is to hold on to the position. Very slow movement engages the muscles for an extended period of time. Holding the muscle in a contracted state keeps the fibers activated. This consumes a lot of energy and results in muscle building.
- Use the interval timer. Vary work and rest intervals. For example, try 20/10 (20 seconds of work+10 seconds of rest) on one day and 50/15 on another day. At the "work" interval, do an exercise as quickly as you can with "as many reps as possible" (AMRAP); during the "rest" interval, rest. Repeat this sequence according to your workout plan.
- Increase the intensity by doing many rounds of exercise or by altering the work/rest interval length.
- Try new exercises. If an exercise sequence gets too easy, your workout will be less effective. That is the time to progress to a more advanced move. There is a huge resource available in books or on the Internet for exercise ideas and techniques if there is no personal trainer available to help you with new

workouts.

- Change your exercise environment. If you usually exercise indoors, try going outdoors. Try working out at a playground, at the beach, or in a field. When you change your environment, you will find new terrain and things to do a new workout with.
- Change the hour of your workout.
- Try new equipment. Best are different types of free weights. These include dumbbells, barbells, clubbells, etc.

A change in workout parameters gives the body added challenge. When there is a challenge, the workouts remain effective.

This book covers only some important exercises. There is, however, an infinite amount of things the human body can do. As long as you focus on building strength, mobility, flexibility, balance, and endurance, you can get creative.

Get inspiration online. The Internet is a great resource for workout routines. Do check out our website for links to exercise routines for all levels.

"It's not the mountain that lies ahead of you that stops you... It's the pebble in your shoe." Muhammad Ali

Work As Hard As You Can

A good attitude pays. Once you have set that amount of time for exercise, do the best you possibly can. Keep your mind focused on building strength, mobility, flexibility, balance, and endurance. Forget about losing weight, because that will naturally happen for you with your new lifestyle.

Think of yourself as a warrior. Tell yourself you're made of great energy. Give your best effort and form for every repetition. Keep your head up. No matter how exhausted you're, stay positive. Complaining and telling yourself you're weak are wasted efforts that will limit the effectiveness of your workout.

Visualize how great you will feel after the session. The harder you work, the better the feeling.

While exercising, put your body in a flow of movements. Enjoy the energy you have in you.

The difference between someone who sees improvement in body

composition and one who goes to the gym for years and doesn't get any fitter is the mind-set one has during the workout sessions. The former sees himself as a warrior with fitness goals to conquer, while the latter is a victim of exhaustion.

If you think like a warrior while working out, you build like a warrior. A victim will look like a victim. Be positive. Think positively. Your mind will give your muscles added energy to move right and grow.

Exercise Will Get Easier with Practice, but Your Workouts Should Stay Challenging

The more you repeat an exercise, the easier it will be to do. That is the time to start doing something different. The body has a tendency to adapt and get used to some exercise routines. No single repetitive exercise can fulfill all goals for the long term. Along the way you will need to do different types of workouts to keep getting better.

Keep going. Every individual is unique. Depending on your workout routine or on whether you get help from a professional, signs of success will appear at different time frames.

Keep your focus. Follow the advice in this chapter.

Most importantly, give yourself time. It may be weeks or months. Just keep working out.

Fitness is a lifestyle; this is a lifelong habit. There is no end point. Keep working out regularly and in the right way, and you will stay forever young, forever fit.

The Mind-Body Connection in Exercise

Exercise is physical activity with a mental connection. When we exercise the body with the right state of consciousness, we're doing it mindfully. Mindfulness during exercise brings great rewards; lack of it results in wasted hours of workouts without observable improvement in physical condition.

There are effectively two extreme kinds of people who say they exercise regularly. The first are those who spend hours at classes or on machines but don't seem to see any significant improvement in their body composition after months of gym membership. Their method of working out is commonly seen in individuals who spend hours running or pounding on treadmills, elliptical machines, or stationary bikes. Another group spends hours in aerobic classes because they are fun. Their reason for working out is usually to "burn calories," "lose weight," or "do some cardio." Most of them are number bound, transfixed on calorie-counting gadgets and heart-rate monitors.

The problem with this attitude toward exercise is that the effect won't last. After months of doing the same exercises, the body gets used to the workout. Since there is no variation, some parts of the body get more developed than others. For example, runners tend to have weak shoulders and arms because few of them care to do push- ups or carry weights.

The other problem with long bouts of cardio, as mentioned earlier, is the burning out of muscles and the wearing out of joints.

When the body gets efficient in doing these exercises, the exerciser gets the sense of getting fit. But the fact is, he is not really getting fit because fitness is not merely about cardiovascular endurance. True fitness is about strength, mobility, flexibility and balance as well.

This is the reason why some people claim they work out but still have problems with fat accumulation.

In the second group are individuals who exercise mindfully and get stunning results (in the form of a lower body fat percentage and an increase in lean body mass) from their workouts. Mindful exercise involves focusing on movement, intensity, and form; doing a variety of exercises; and putting in maximum effort at each session, with the goal of becoming truly fit (in other words, building muscle for strength, mobility, flexibility, balance, and endurance.). This way of exercising brings observable improvement to physique and ultimately to youthfulness.

The difference between the two groups is in their extent of mindfulness when they exercise. You would want to be a member of the second team. While all kinds of exercises will work in the immediate term, most random workout routines will not work for the long term. This is a phenomenon called "hitting the plateau." That is because the human body has a way of getting used to repetitive exercises.

MINDFUL EXERCISE	REPETITIVE EXERCISE
Focus on movement and form	Focus on numbers
Builds strength, mobility, fexibility, endurance, balance -- Fitness	"Fat Burning"
Intensity	Time
Variation	Repetitive
Full body focus	No focus on body
Results in muscle building, tissue and bone regeneration	Burns fat and other tissues
Gain muscle mass, increase RMR	Lose muscle mass, decrease RMR
Short workout sessions	Long workout sessions

Workouts for any reason other than building strength, mobility, flexibility, and endurance are not going to get you really fit.

On the flip side, when you do exercise mindfully, you get the maximum benefit for your efforts. Your body will be leaner, stronger, and more flexible. You will find performing daily tasks to be easier. You will feel more energetic, more in the mood to take part in spontaneous activity. That kind of approach to exercise will give you real, long-lasting fitness.

Do not become number bound.

Don't fall into the trap of getting number bound. Numbers are pure illusions that don't reflect real human physiology.

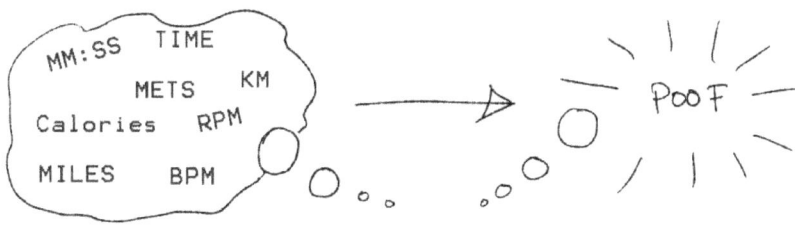

Forget numbers while exercising

Exercise becomes more effective when the mind is free of numbers and more focused on how the body moves.

The human body is not an inanimate engine but a complex machine that runs on closely regulated biochemical reactions.

You don't "burn" six hundred calories simply because the treadmill says so. Exercise machines are created with gimmickry to make the user reliant on it with the purpose to sell more exercise machines.

The same is true for heart-rate monitors. If you learn how to feel your body during your workout, you will know when you've reached your maximum heart rate.

Estimate the level of your workout with a 0 to 10 scale. This scale is an estimation of the level of exertion during exercise.

Exertion - heart rate & breathing during exercise:

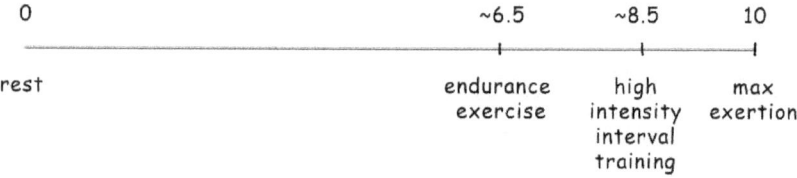

Feeling of muscle discomfort during exercise:

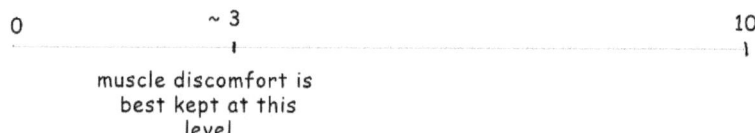

Learning how to feel your body is an important step. You have to know your potential and your limits. There is such a thing as under exercising and over exercising, both of which would not bring the full benefits of the exercise.

You can use the technique of perceived exertion to gauge the intensity of exercise. It is an arbitrary scale of zero to ten, with zero being how you feel at the point of rest and ten being how you would feel at the point of complete exertion.

Learning to feel your body will free you from being bound to numbers. This freedom will make the workouts more effective in attaining your true fitness goals.

Fitness is the Best Purpose for Exercise

Exercise is a double-edged sword. It is like a risky investment. How well you benefit from the time you put aside for your workouts will determine the extent of your success.

Be aware that exercise can be a time-wasting, self-destructive activity if done with the wrong focus—for example, like the focus on mindlessly burning away calories. Burning calories without building muscles ages the body and does nothing to improve overall fitness.

Effective exercise is different because it is done with the right mind-set—with the constant focus on getting fit. Exercise with this kind of attitude will bring long-lasting rewards.

Work out regularly with the aim of gaining the five attributes of fitness—strength, mobility, flexibility, balance, and endurance. You will find your body getting healthier, leaner, and more youthful.

Physical vitality has a profound influence in all other aspects of your life. You will feel more confident, happy, and self-sustaining.

Chapter 5: Food, Glorious Food

Food is the source of all the nutrients our bodies need to stay forever young and fit. In a world where food is often demonized as the cause of obesity and illness, it is easy to forget that we actually need to eat well to stay alive. This chapter is extensive because lots of facts about nutrition need clarification. To be able to eat right, we must know nutritional science.

We shall focus on the importance of getting the right nutrients from the food we eat by

- discussing the macro and micronutrients and their role in building, maintaining, and replenishing physiological structure and function;
- laying to rest common diet myths;
- doing away with fad diets;
- doing away with calorie counting and starvation; and
- learning how to make good nutrition a natural lifestyle choice.

What is food really? Everything we eat, be it the finest-quality filet steak or a hamburger at a fast-food joint, ultimately gets broken down into its basic building blocks in our digestive system. The nutrients derived from digestion can be very simply categorized by the relative quantities that exist in nature—the macronutrients and micronutrients.

Macronutrients, or "macros," make up the bulk of the dry weight in foods. These are all organic in nature and include carbohydrates, proteins, and fats. Their molecules are large, complex building blocks, which are materially essential for the structure and form of all living organisms. Carbohydrates and fats are also the main energy source for living cells.

Our bodies need micronutrients, or "micros," in small quantities. These are the important substances that are necessary for biochemical reactions to take place effectively within living cells. Micronutrients include organic compounds such as vitamins, phytochemicals, and inorganic compounds like mineral salts.

Organs, Tissues and Cells

The body is made up of organs like the brain, heart, lungs, skin and so forth. These organs are made up of tissues like muscle tissues and liver tissues, or the connective tissues that encase the organs keeping them in shape. These tissues are made up of specialized cells. For example liver cells are found in liver tissue, and muscle fibers are specialized cells only found in the muscles. The cells are units of life. These cells are made of proteins, fat and some components of carbohydrates. The cell are also connected together by intercellular material, which is made up of mostly protein.

Cells, being living units, need constant supply of nutrients for function and energy. Cells also die and get replaced. These processes require nutrients that have to come from our diet.

Protein Builds Life

Our lean body mass (mass of the body excluding the excess fat mass) contains about 21 percent protein. Protein can be considered the building block of life. The function of protein in every living organism is the following:

•   Structure. We all know protein is an important component of muscle cells and hence movement. Protein is also the structural component of tissues in the body—from the tendons that link the muscles to bones; to connective tissues that hold the organs in shape; to collagen that make up skin; to hair, nails, and even parts of bone.

•   Cell (biochemical) function. Smaller protein molecules such as enzymes, hormones, organic cofactors, cell receptors, neurotransmitters, carriers, and biochemically active compounds are important molecules that help along all the biochemical processes in the cells of the body.

•   Viscosity of blood and fluid in cells.

Protein molecules are chains of amino-acids linked together by peptide bonds. The unique sequence of amino-acids create the specific protein structure.

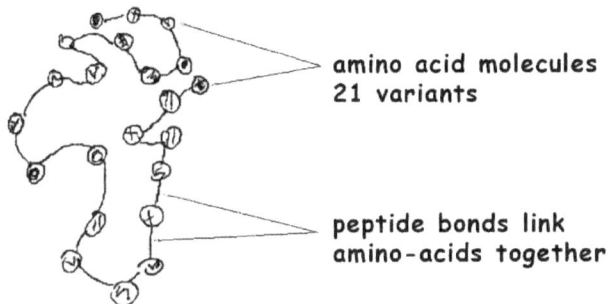

amino acid molecules
21 variants

peptide bonds link
amino-acids together

Proteins are large molecules made up of building blocks called amino acids. Combinations of twenty-one amino acids make up all the proteins in the human body. Of these twenty-one amino acids, twelve can be produced by the body itself, and nine are not produced by the body and must come from our food source.

These nine amino acids are called "essential amino acids." Amino acids, especially the nine essential amino acids, are important components for a healthy, complete diet. Amino acids are building units of protein for the structure and function of cells in tissues and organs. Cells in our bodies make the required protein according to the information and signals given by genetic material (DNA). Each protein molecule must have the amino acids strung up in an exact combination to be functional.

Amino acids also have complex roles as neurotransmitters (the chemicals that send messages between nerve cells) and help in building up other important biological compounds. Long-term deficiency in amino acids will result in the degeneration of health and accelerated aging.

Plants and animal sources of food contain protein. The most complete sources of amino acids, however, come from animal protein: meat, poultry, fish, and eggs. Animal products are easily digestible, and animal protein contains all the amino acids necessary for healthy body function.

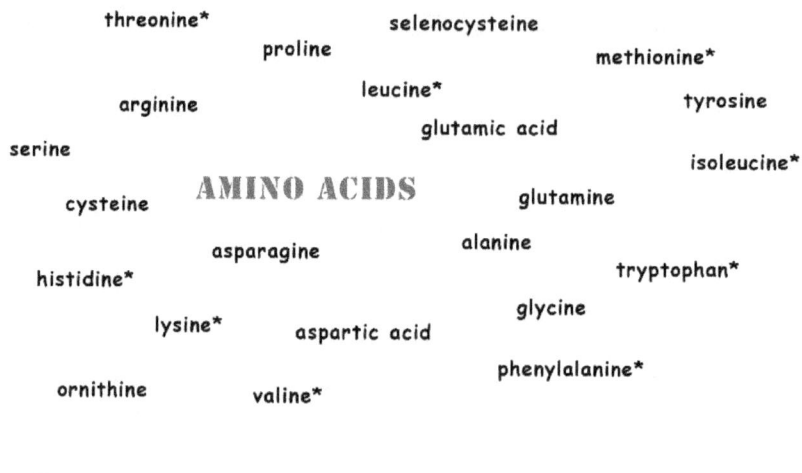

*essential amino acids

Beyond the nutritional benefits of consuming adequate amounts of protein in our diets, there is an added plus to eating protein at mealtime. That is obesity control. Proteins take more energy to digest than refined carbohydrates, sugar, and alcohol do. Proteins in the diet contribute less to net calorie input than carbohydrates do.

Proteins also tend to stay in the stomach longer than refined carbohydrates. Research has shown that proteins leave us feeling satisfied faster and longer, so we're less likely to snack or even overeat.

Proteins in the diet don't induce insulin surges we get after a carbohydrate-rich meal, which means that there is no likelihood of excessive fat accumulation and no hindrance to fat burning. There is more discussion about insulin effects in the section on carbohydrate metabolism in this chapter.

Plan Your Meals Around a Protein Source

There is no hard-and-fast rule as to how much protein we should consume at each meal. We should not get number bound and start counting and weighing. The easiest rule to follow is that the protein component of food should take priority. Make sure there is enough protein on your plate. Even when you snack, make sure there is protein in the snack.

Another strategy to get more protein into your diet is to eat the protein component first. If you eat all the protein on your plate first, there will be less space in the stomach for nutrient-poor carbohydrates that might be there.

Plan your meals around protein. Good protein sources in common foods include the following:

- Eggs
- Poultry
- Lean cuts of beef
- Lean cuts of pork
- Fish (oily fish is actually good for you)
- Shellfish
- Protein-rich vegetables like legumes and nuts

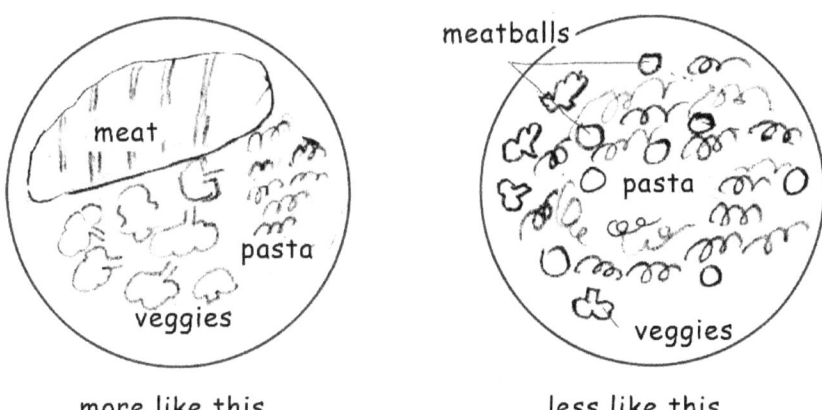

more like this   less like this

Protein, not carbs, should be main part of the dish.

The above protein-rich whole foods should make up the bulk of your meal. This means you have enough of these protein sources to satisfy hunger. Have the vegetables, fats, and carbohydrates on the side. Planning meals this way is the secret to getting enough proteins for prolonged health and fitness.

Fat is Not the Enemy

The human body has two categories of fat:

- Storage fat. Storage fat is the excess fat stored under the skin in tissues called adipose tissues. This excess fat is harmless and needed during Paleolithic (stone-age) times to survive famine. Nowadays, of course, fat in the adipose tissues is regarded as a nuisance because it makes us look flabby, something to be "burned off." This is the fat we understand as the indicator of obesity. Depending on individuals, the percentage of storage fat varies significantly.

- Essential fat. Essential fat is necessary fat for human survival. Essential fat percentage in men is 7 percent and in women is 12 percent.

What is the function of fat in the body? Every cell in the body is made up of at least 2 percent fat. Nerve and brain cells contain more fat. Fats in the cells and body fluids are called "lipids." Lipids make up the cell structure. Without lipids, the cell would not exist.

- Fat is an essential stored-energy source. If the diet is right, fat is the body's preferred source of energy.
- Some internal organs are protected by fatty tissue, which acts as a cushion and support.
- Fat is a carrier to transport essential chemicals and hormones for biological function.
- Fat is a lubricant in organs.
- Free fatty acids in cells and the bloodstream are used as fuel to build and modify protein and for producing other compounds like neurotransmitters (molecules responsible for nerve function).

When we take fat out of our food, we become deficient in the following nutrients:

- Essential fatty acids like omega-3 fatty acids and omega-6 fatty acids. These are building blocks of cells and factors needed for cell function.
- Vitamins like vitamins A, D, E, and K which can only dissolve in fat (fat-soluble vitamins) and other lipid-soluble compounds. These vitamins need fat, not water, as a solvent so they can be transported into the blood. Low-fat or non-fat food lack these vitamins.

A diet deficient in fat means a deficiency in essential nutrients. This leads to degeneration and deterioration of the body, which is a primer for accelerated aging and chronic illnesses.

We need fat in our diets. Good fat sources include olive oil, fish, nuts and seeds, avocado, coconut, and eggs.

Eating Fat Alone Will Not Make You Fat

Refined carbohydrates, including sugar, in our diets cause obesity, not dietary fat. Processed, low-fat foods are no healthy option!

Those who cook often understand the importance of fat to the taste and look of cooked food.

A home-baked pound cake, for example, made without butter will turn out crumbly, dry, and rock hard. If you try to make nonfat yogurt with skimmed milk, you'll get an unappetizing, lumpy product. Fat makes food delicious because it is a carrier for aromatic molecules that make food smell and taste great. Fat also gives food its creamy sensation in the mouth by lingering on the tongue.

To create their factory-made "fat-free" versions of food, the food industry replaces fat with refined starches and gels. This step compensates for the loss in the appeal of the food when fat is absent. When you substitute your full-fat foods for the low-fat variety, you actually increase your refined carbohydrate intake.

Diets dominated by refined carbohydrates, as we will discuss later, are a cause of obesity, aging, and age-related illnesses. Fat, on the other hand, is an important nutrient.

There is really no good reason to choose low-fat versions of packaged foods over regular, full-fat foods.

Fats are fatty-acid molecules linked together by a glycerol head to form a Tri-glyceride molecule

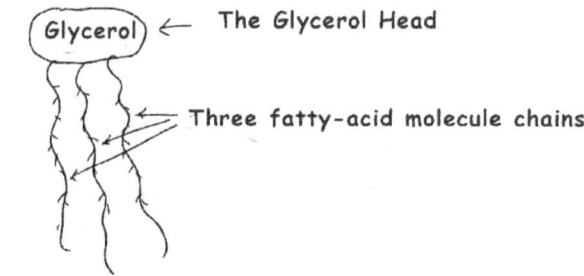

Tri-glyceride Molecule

Good Fat vs. Bad Fat

Foods that contain good fats are rich in essential fatty acids like omega-3 fatty acids. They also contain fat-soluble vitamins. Essential fatty acids are, as the term implies, important for a wide range of biological functions.

There is also such a thing as "bad fat" or unhealthy fat. These are the fats to avoid. These are trans fats.

Trans fats are human-engineered fats that can be found in highly processed baked, roasted foods; fried foods; and hydrogenated cooking oil. These fats are engineered to be more heat stable, enabling the food to be cooked more quickly. And since these fats are almost indestructible, they give processed foods a longer shelf life.

Trans fats can be found in meats but in much smaller quantities than in processed foods.

Trans fats wreak havoc upon entering the bloodstream, causing inflammation, clogging arteries, and leading to common chronic ailments.

The good news is that the world is slowly coming to grips with the harmful effects of trans fats. More governments are getting tough on its use in food.

As far as fat in your diet is concerned, it is better to choose whole unprocessed foods that are rich in natural, good fats. These foods contain essential nutrients that are present in the fat necessary for health. Here are some healthy tips:

- Always have olive oil, nuts, seeds, and avocado available in your kitchen.
- Eat oily fish, meats, and eggs.
- Choose whole-fat dairy rather than the low-fat option.
- Avoid processed, baked, fried, and roasted snacks as well as margarine and spreads that may contain trans fat.

If you have been avoiding all fat in your diet, it is time to change. Replace refined carbohydrates in your diet with food that is rich in protein and good fat. Eat the "good" fats without fear. You need essential fatty acids for cell function. Cells are the basic units of tissues and organs.

Having enough good fat sources in your diet will supply the body with all the essential fatty acids and vitamins you need. This is a positive way to help you stay young and healthy.

Carbohydrates: The Good and the Ugly

Carbohydrates are a source of energy for the human body. We consume them from plant sources and milk. Meats and eggs don't contain significant amounts of carbohydrate.

Carbohydrates are large molecules of reducing sugar units linked together. There are three types of reducing sugars naturally found in our diets:

- Glucose is the most common one and a component of all starches. Glucose is the universal fuel every cell in the human body uses. Because of its importance in metabolism, the glucose level in the blood is kept at a constant level by the hormone insulin. This is a very significant fact, which we shall discuss further in this chapter.
- Fructose is found naturally in plants. Due to its taste and sweetness, fructose is also used as an additive in our food and drinks. Table sugar, or sucrose, and high-fructose corn syrup (HFCS) are high sources of fructose in our diets. While fructose is a fuel source, overconsumption of this sugar has

harmful effects on our health.

- Galactose is found naturally in milk and some plants. It is most commonly found in our diets as lactose.

Carbohydrate molecules are large structures made up of smaller sugar molecules

Simple Sugar (one sugar molecule)
Glucose, Fructose and Galactose

Disaccharides (two sugar molecules)
Sucrose, Lactose, Maltose

Polysaccharides (usually 200-2500 glucose molecules)
Amylose, Amylopectin

Carbohydrates in the digested form enter the bloodstream as simple sugars. Disaccharides like sucrose break down into glucose and fructose, while polysaccharides break down into glucose molecules.

Simple sugars are single molecules of sugar. These molecules, which can move freely in the body via blood and other intracellular fluids, are also highly reactive. While being useful for cell metabolism in regulated quantities, they can cause damage to organs and cell structures.

Excess glucose is removed through a regulatory mechanism that involves the hormone insulin. Where possible, glucose in the blood gets taken up by the cells in the body for metabolism, a process in which glucose molecules is broken down to carbon dioxide and water to produce energy. Excess glucose gets stored in the liver and muscles as larger carbohydrate molecules called glycogen. The glycogen storage in the human body is very limited. Further excess of glucose gets converted to fat by the liver. This fat is transported to the adipose tissues for storage.

There is no biological regulation in the body for fructose and galactose. These sugars are removed from the bloodstream only via the liver.

The Insulin Connection

Insulin is a hormone that functions to regulate the concentration of glucose in the blood and body fluids. While glucose is a fuel source for all cells in the body, it is also a harmful substance when consumed in excess. We must therefore keep the level of blood glucose at a constant level.

Glucose, fructose, and galactose are classified as reducing sugars. Reducing sugars are highly reactive molecules that bond spontaneously with protein and lipid molecules in a chemical reaction called glycation, which causes damage to the larger molecules. The resulting damaged protein or fat molecule is called advanced glycation end products (AGEs). The consequence of this damage is the breakdown in structure of cells and tissue.

Glycation of Protein

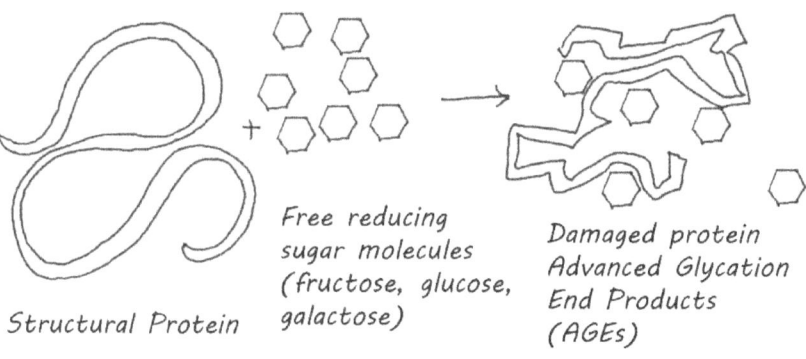

Structural Protein

Free reducing sugar molecules (fructose, glucose, galactose)

Damaged protein Advanced Glycation End Products (AGEs)

The toxic effects of glucose can commonly be seen in sufferers of untreated diabetes. The blood glucose levels in these individuals are constantly high. Free glucose molecules in high concentrations attack cellular structures, causing organ damage. Symptoms include blindness, neurological problems, stroke, and heart disease.

Glucose enters the bloodstream from the intestine as a result of digested carbohydrate and sugar. An increase in glucose concentration in the blood triggers insulin production. Insulin acts to mop up excess glucose by a number of processes:

- Storing glucose in the liver and muscle as glycogen. There is a limit as to how much glycogen can be stored. In general

it is about five hundred grams in a standard human body.
- Converting excess glucose to fat
- Suppressing fat from being metabolized. In other words, fat burning is hindered since glucose in the blood must be used first.

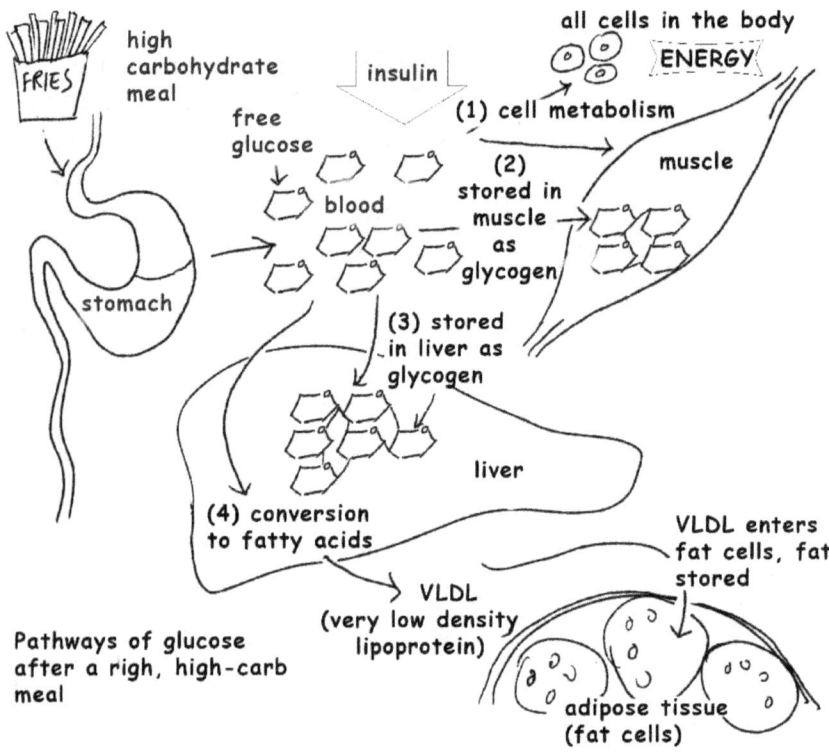

Pathways of glucose after a righ, high-carb meal

There is a dangerous limit. The modern diet is high in refined carbohydrates. Every time we have a meal loaded with carbohydrates, blood glucose concentration goes up and insulin levels spike. Insulin is like a signaling device that activates different cells in the body to mop up excess glucose in the blood.

Constant insulin secretion has these consequences:
- Hunger swings. Hypoglycemia is a situation where blood-

glucose levels dive to an uncomfortable low. When this happens—usually less than two hours after a carbohydrate-loaded meal—we get tired and hungry. Hence the hunger swings, the carbohydrate cravings, and the vicious cycle of overeating.

There is a reason why carbohydrate-rich foods are highly addictive. Carbohydrate-laden foods affect pleasure sensors in the brain. Different carbohydrate sources affect the brain differently. That is why our "comfort food" lists commonly consist of these high-carbohydrate sources.

- Fat storing. Unlike plants, the human body has only limited capacity to store carbohydrates. Excess sugar in the blood has to be converted to fat for storage in the adipose tissues. The consequence is, of course, obesity.
- Fat sparing. Consistently high blood sugar and constant insulin spikes cause fat not only to build up but also to be locked in. Insulin signals all the cells in the body to prefer glucose as fuel since it has become readily available in the blood. As a result, the machinery for fat burning slows. This leads to fat build up and the difficulty to lose fat even with exercise.

When we're in the habit of consuming consistently high amounts of refined carbohydrates, our bodies learn to burn glucose as a main source of energy. We get hungry when the available glucose runs low. This happens very quickly since glucose doesn't stay in the blood of a non-diabetic person for very long.

A body that is running predominantly on glucose and is constantly secreting insulin will store up fat because fat is not its fuel of choice.

When the body is unable to use its fat stores, it runs out of energy very quickly, since insulin keeps glucose at a low level. This leaves the person feeling fatigued, lacking in energy, and in need of eating more carbohydrate-rich food.

It is a vicious cycle. The only way to break the cycle is to cut out refined carbohydrates as the main source of food—or cut it out completely, if possible.

The eventual system breakdown in the system caused by over consuming refined carbohydrates results in insulin resistance or type 2 diabetes. Cells in the body will cease to respond to insulin. This makes insulin function useless.

Those who don't suffer from diabetes might see the effects of overconsumption of carbohydrate-rich foods manifest as the following:

- Obesity
- Premature signs of aging
- Hypertension
- Cardiovascular disease
- Cancers
- Nerve- and muscle-coordination problems

We can reduce and eliminate these health risks by setting our minds on fully understanding carbohydrates in our diets.

Bad Carbohydrates, Good Carbohydrates and the Glycemic Index

Not all carbohydrate sources are alike. There are the bad and the good. Bad carbohydrate sources include foods that cause blood sugar levels in the blood to rise quickly on digestion.

The effect of bad sources of carbohydrates includes the following:

- They cause a sudden increase in blood sugar. This rise forces insulin to spike, contributing to a chain of biochemical reactions in the body that are responsible for obesity.
- They contain no or very little micronutrients. Consuming these sources of carbohydrates puts excess energy into our bodies without providing any other essential nutrients. It is what we call "empty calories." Excess energy converts to fat.
- They lead to the consumption of empty calories, resulting in a condition of malnourishment accompanied by obesity. Malnourishment leads to the degenerative process of aging. This is the reason why someone can get fat while the organs in the body starve until they become sick.
- They contain no or very little fiber. Fiber slows down the absorption of glucose into the blood, keeping its concentration at a safe level. The only way to get enough fiber is to consume whole vegetables and fruit.

We mostly find examples of bad carbohydrate sources in processed food, including the following:

- Refined flour-based foods like breads, cakes, pastries, and biscuits, including their whole-grain versions
- Sauces and dressings containing starch, flour, and sugar

- Jams and preserves
- Candy or confectionery
- Soft drinks, fruit juices, and sugared beverages
- Noodles and pasta
- Sweet desserts
- Starchy vegetables like potatoes
- Grains like rice, oats, and barley
- Breakfast cereals
- Low-fat dairy products that may contain starch additives

These are foods that are likely to have high glycemic index (GI). The glycemic index (GI) is a scale of 0 to 100 that ranks foods according to the extent to which they raise blood-glucose levels in the blood relative to pure glucose, which ranks one hundred. We can find information about food and their corresponding GI values online.

We're advised to choose food with the lower GI option to control our blood-glucose levels.

While GI values provide good guidance, they are only a measurement to rate glucose absorption in the blood from ingesting food. It is not a measure of the sugar fructose. Pure fructose has a GI value in the range of ten, and it is not a healthy source of carbohydrates.

We also need to be aware that GI measures only the rate of absorption and not the absolute amount of carbohydrates in food. That is called the glycemic load (GL). GL takes into account both GI and the total number of carbohydrates in a serving of a particular food.

Overeating low GI foods with high GL can also lead to excess fat storage due to excess carbohydrates in the diet—although that is not as bad as consuming foods with a high GI and GL.

The best way to deal with all this is to analyze available lists of GI and GL values of the food you commonly eat. Make your own lists of foods you should eat more of and those you will abstain from.

Choose rightly. Avoid all processed, refined carbohydrates, starchy vegetables, and grains.

Get your carbohydrates instead from green leafy vegetables, roots, stems, and flowers of vegetables—with the exception of starchy tubers like potatoes, mushrooms, whole fruits, nuts, seeds, and legumes.

It would be best to consume minimally processed vegetables—either raw or lightly cooked. Fresh vegetables contain life-enhancing micronutrients that keep better with less cooking.

Soluble fiber in plant tissue forms tiny barriers that hinder digestive enzymes in the small intestines from getting to the carbohydrates. This process slows down digestion and the absorption of sugars into the bloodstream (lower Glycemic Index).

Incidentally, the fibers in whole grains don't reduce the GI because these non-soluble fibers don't form effective barriers against digestive enzymes.

Get your carbohydrates from the right food sources.

 How many carbohydrates one should eat depends on one's physical activity level, since most excess calories from carbohydrates get stored as fat.

Is Sugar a Poison?

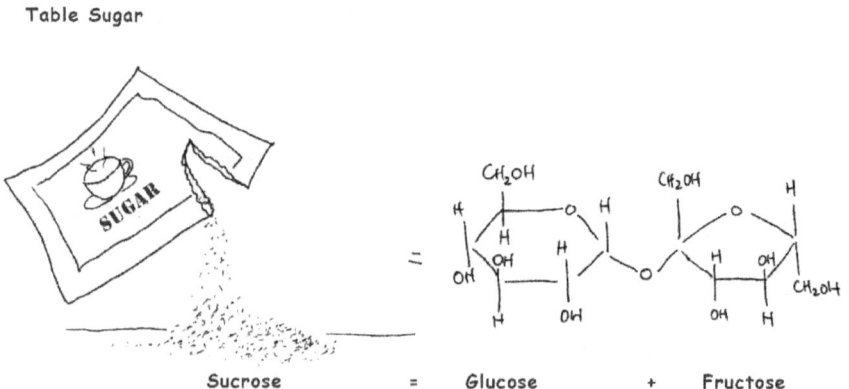

Table Sugar

Sucrose   =   Glucose   +   Fructose

When we talk about sugar, the additive we use to sweeten everything, we're referring to a molecule called sucrose. Sucrose is a glucose-fructose disaccharide. When we consume sugar, free glucose and fructose enter the bloodstream.

Glucose, we know, is a molecule all cells in the body use for energy. The hormone insulin regulates it in the blood. Fructose doesn't affect the secretion of insulin and can only be processed in the liver. Therefore, the GI of sucrose is in the range of 60 percent.

The metabolic pathway of fructose is similar to that of alcohol.

Both can be processed only by the liver.

If we compare the above diagram with the processing of glucose, we observe the difference:

While some of the absorbed glucose gets used up by other cells in the body and even stored in muscles, fructose gets used only when it enters the liver. This means that all fructose entering the bloodstream needs to be processed by liver cells, to remove it from the body.

Fructose level is not moderated in the body. No hormone like insulin is secreted in response to high-fructose blood levels.

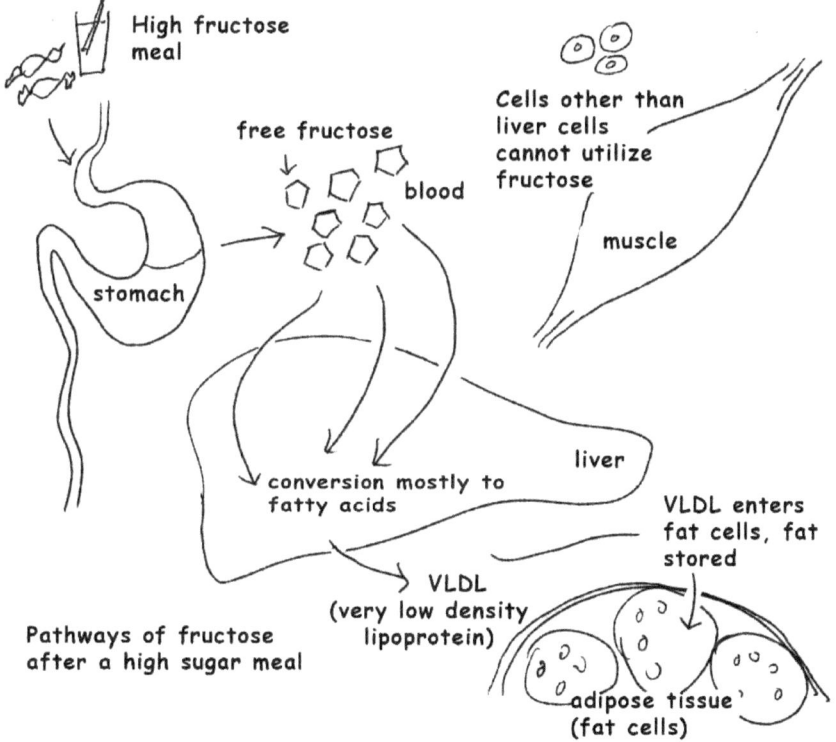

High fructose meal

free fructose

blood

Cells other than liver cells cannot utilize fructose

muscle

stomach

conversion mostly to fatty acids

liver

VLDL enters fat cells, fat stored

VLDL (very low density lipoprotein)

Pathways of fructose after a high sugar meal

adipose tissue (fat cells)

What are the health repercussions of long-term overconsumption of fructose?

- Leptin resistance. Leptin is a hormone that gives us the sensation of satiety, which means a sensation of being not hungry anymore. It normally kicks in twenty minutes after the start of a meal. Fructose has been known to suppress the effects of leptin, thereby causing us to keep eating.
- Obesity, since the body converts excess fructose to fat.
- Type 2 diabetes, metabolic syndrome, whereby the body

cannot regulate sugar in the blood. While fructose doesn't trigger insulin secretion in the body, some have hypothesized that it is a cause of insulin resistance, a condition where the cells in the body cannot respond to insulin anymore, leading to metabolic syndrome.

- Cardiovascular disease and stroke, since excess fructose exits the liver as VLDL (Very Low Density Lipoprotein). VLDL is a precursor to more LDL (Low Density Lipoprotein), which are the components of plaques that get deposited in the arteries.
- Damage to tissue by glycation. This is most observable in skin and bone damage. The symptoms are akin to premature aging, because the cellular structures in the body get damaged in the process.
- Gout due to increased uric acid (a waste-product of fructose processing in the liver) deposited from the metabolism of fructose
- Nonalcoholic fatty liver disease. Overconsumption of fructose will overload the functions of the liver, thereby causing symptoms of fatty liver and liver tissue damage.

Sugar addiction poses the same health risks as alcoholism. The mechanics by which the body metabolizes alcohol (in its digested state, it is called ethanol) are similar to the way it metabolizes fructose. The key difference between consuming fructose and consuming alcohol is that fructose doesn't bring the sensation of drunkenness. Just because fructose doesn't intoxicate, put us on a high, or cause us to be merry, throw up, pass out, or get a hangover, that doesn't make it safer to consume than alcohol. Since there is no warning of an overdose, fructose is actually a more harmful substance.

Like alcohol, fructose is also very addictive. That is why it is very difficult for most of us who are used to having sugary drinks, sweets, chocolates, and other snacks to completely quit eating them.

Large quantities of fructose in our diets come from the following:

- Table sugar, soft drinks, sweetened drinks
- Fruit juices
- Baked goods,
- Confectionery
- Desserts
- Jams and preserves
- Sauces

- Natural sweeteners like honey and maple syrup
- Processed foods, sauces, and salad dressings
- Breakfast cereals
- Sweetened milk products
- Dried fruit
- Fresh whole fruit – fruit in its natural form, cut or pureed but not juiced, sweetened or extracted in any way.

Of all the items in the above list, whole fresh or dried fruit is the only safe source of fructose we can eat in abundance. Soluble fiber in the fruit hinders the absorption of fructose in the small intestines, slowing down the process to a safe level. Fruits also have micronutrients important for body functions, making them a reasonable payoff. Even so, we should consume fruit only in its whole form, not juiced, with moderation.

If you want to experience a 180-degree turn in your health for the better, see immediate loss of excess fat in your body, and alleviate aging-related disease symptoms, cut down on your sugar intake for good.

- Drink nothing that contains added sugar, such as soft drinks, energy drinks, and sweetened drinks.
- Drink no juices.
- Eat fruit whole in moderation.
- Eat very little amounts of desserts, cakes, or confectionery.

Stay away from any processed food that has added sugar, fructose, glucose syrup, or high-fructose corn syrup.

- Avoid natural sweeteners like honey, maple syrup, treacle, and so forth.
- Avoid dairy products that contain sugar.

If you find that cutting back on sweets and fructose-containing foods is very restrictive and difficult to do, this is only because sugar is addictive. The best way to stop addiction is to understand that things will get easier if you just stick to the process of breaking the habit. You can do the following:

- Go to your kitchen and discard all sources of sugar. It is all right to throw away food items that are more harmful than nutritious. Grab a garbage bag and toss away all sugar, chocolate mixes, candy, frozen muffins, ketchup, and so forth.
- Make a list of all the foods you will not buy from the grocery store anymore. That is easy enough. Then make sure you don't

go shopping on an empty stomach.
- Think of all the healthy foods you should eat instead and stock the kitchen only with those. If you're used to munching on potato chips in front of the TV, buy a bag of oven-roasted mixed nuts instead. That is not a perfect solution, but it is a good start to wean you off refined carbohydrate snacks.

If you failed to meet your goals and binge on a sweet or two, don't despair. This is a lifelong habit change. Think positively and get back on the right track.

How to Keep Excess Fat Off by Eating Right

Fat is an excellent fuel source for most tissues in the body. The breakdown of fatty acid molecules by cells releases a chemical called ATP (Adenosine Tri-phosphate). Production of ATP and its role in providing energy to cells is a complex process. All we need to understand now is that fat breakdown provides the cells with ATP which is energy for activities such as:
- Movement (in muscles)
- Heat production
- Biochemical functions like cell growth, wound healing, and so forth

Apart from the brain, which needs glucose for fuel, most cells in the body can burn fat for energy. When we have enough fuel, we will feel energetic. When our fuel source runs low, however, we will automatically feel lethargic and hungry.

Most of us today have excess fat stored in our adipose tissues that lie under the skin. This being the case, we should feel energetic, but we don't. Some of us even feel hungry all the time, when in theory the energy in stored fat should keep us going for hours, even days.

We feel deprived of energy because the cells in our bodies that should burn fat are not burning fat effectively. This is caused by the lingering presence of insulin in the blood.

Insulin, by acting to clear up glucose from blood, signals all cells to prefer glucose as a fuel source. When cells start metabolizing glucose instead of metabolizing fat, fat gets locked up in the adipose tissues and made unavailable as fuel for the metabolism.

Another way to understand this is to imagine two switches one can flip so cells get energy: the glucose-burning switch and the fat-burning switch. Only one switch is allowed to be turned on at a time. Normally the fat-burning switch is turned on. Fat is an innate fuel of choice for most cells because it is a form of fuel the body can store in good amounts. Glucose, on the other hand, runs out quickly because it is stored in very limited amounts as glycogen in the liver and muscles.

If glucose levels are high via regular high-carbohydrate diets, the glucose-metabolizing switch is turned on, and the fat-metabolizing switch is turned off due to the influence of insulin.

The process of turning switches on and off takes weeks. Though it sounds like a simple idea, it is actually a complex regulatory process whereby genes are activated to produce enzymes for the respective fuel-utilizing machinery.

Control the amount of carbohydrate-rich foods in your diet to relieve your body from having to deal with the constant onslaught of glucose in the blood. This will result in metabolic changes in which the body will readjust its fuel choice naturally—to burn fat instead of glucose. When you change your diet this way, it will take about one hundred days to realize an improvement in your fat-utilizing capability.

The other effect of insulin, as mentioned earlier, is that it converts excess sugars into fat. This further increases fat stored in fat cells. If the body is switched on to burn glucose—while excess glucose that enters the blood is stored as fat—more fat gets stored up and locked away in adipose tissues. When glucose is converted to fat, there is no more fuel source for the cells that want only glucose as fuel. The result is a feeling of fatigue and hunger. When we get fatigued, we move less. When hunger strikes and we consume more carbohydrate-rich foods, the fat-storing cycle continues.

Listen to your body. Are you hungry for carbohydrates? Do you suffer lack of energy between meals? Do you suffer hunger swings? Are you putting on fat despite exercise and diets? Take refined carbohydrates out of your diet. The beginning of a new diet low in refined carbohydrates might be an uncomfortable experience, with feelings of fatigue and mood swings. The body needs a bit of time to change the switch—from glucose metabolizing to fat metabolizing, to unlock fat stores and to burn fat. Keep it up. Be patient and hang in there.

So, What's For Breakfast?

The traditional breakfast menu for most of us in the developed world is dominated by refined carbohydrates. The first meal of our day usually centers on breads, cereals, pancakes, pastries, sugary dairy drinks, fruit juices, and so forth. These foods, consumed in abundance, will ultimately enter the blood as simple sugars. This triggers the secretion of insulin, followed by a cascade of biochemical events that manifest in the short term as hunger swings and in the long term as fat accumulation. Reduce your intake of refined carbohydrate foods by starting each day with more nutritious, low-carbohydrate alternatives such as the following:

- Eggs—boiled, poached, served sunny side up, scrambled, served in omelet form
- Vegetables—non-starchy types, mushrooms
- Strips of lean chicken, beef, pork or venison, spiced with a thin strip of bacon
- Cheese (the natural, full-fat variety)
- Mixed nuts and seeds (raw or dry roasted is best)
- Avocado
- A serving of whole fruit

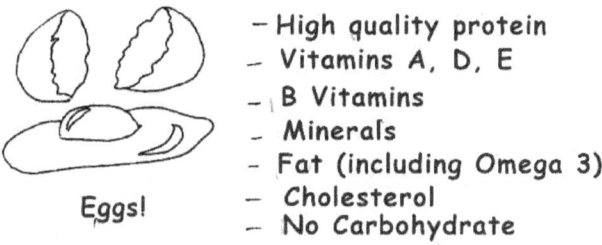

Eggs!

– High quality protein
– Vitamins A, D, E
– B Vitamins
– Minerals
– Fat (including Omega 3)
– Cholesterol
– No Carbohydrate

Eggs? This sounds like the opposite of our conventional idea of a "healthy low-fat breakfast," right? Yes it is, because low fat is not the healthy option. The idea that eating grain-based food is healthy is also a myth. Grains like wheat, barley, oats, and rice, including the whole grain varieties, are high in easily digestible carbohydrates. Consuming stacks of bread, pancakes, and rice porridge will just send your blood glucose levels up.

If you must eat grain-based foods for breakfast, be aware of the effect they will have on your metabolism. Reduce the portions of these foods and replace them with low-carbohydrate alternatives.

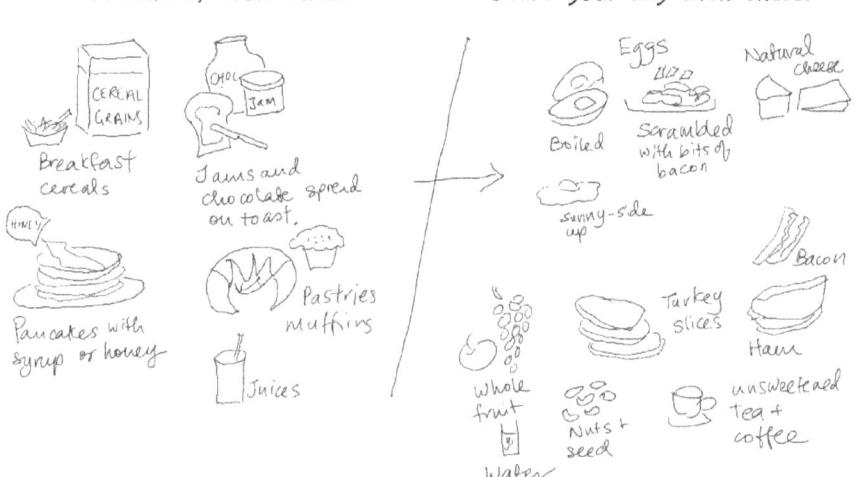

At breakfast, avoid these: *Start your day with these:*

You don't need to eat less, just eat differently.

Try this yourself for a month. You will notice a difference in the way your body looks and feels.

Water and the Fountain of Youth

Mentioning the dietary importance of water is almost a cliché. We all know this, but many of us still don't drink enough. It could be that water drinking isn't interesting and can sometimes be inconvenient. Water is our most important dietary component because almost 70 percent of our body mass is water.

Water has these functions:

•   Water creates bulk in all living cells. Lack of water (or dehydration) causes cells to lose their mass, get deformed, and eventually die. As a result, tissues and organs get damaged.

•   Water is the universal solvent. Water dissolves gases, mineral ions (salts), vitamins, toxins, and other organic and inorganic substances. These chemicals and biochemicals need to be dissolved in water for essential chemical interactions to occur.

•   Water is a transporter. Large organic molecules—for example, lipoproteins, enzymes, hormones, neurotransmitters, and cells like blood cells—need to move around the body. Moving liquid in the body is predominantly water. It is like a river that needs to stay fluid. When dry, the river will not allow boats carrying cargo to pass from one location to the next.

- Water maintains the internal environment of the body in a process called homeostasis (*homo* means "the same" or "constant", and *stasis* means "to stand still"). Homeostasis is a process where the fluids in the body is always kept within a fixed conditions.

Tissues and organs are very sensitive to change in its environmental parameters, which include body temperature, acidity, electrolytes and solutes, sugar, blood pressure, and so forth. These parameters have to be kept constant. The cardiovascular system keeps blood and body fluids in constant flow so that the regulatory measure initiated by an organ like the liver is transported to the whole body.

Water facilitates cell-to-cell communication. Cells in different organs and tissues communicate via neurotransmission and hormone secretion. These communication processes require fluids in the body.

How Much Water is Enough?

Your daily water requirement depends on several factors: for example, the climate you're in, your activity level, the food you eat. As with everything else, there is no need to get number bound and start counting the number of glasses to drink per day. It is just best to drink little sips of water throughout the day. Have a glass before and after each meal. Carry a bottle of water around with you every time you engage in physical activity. Drink more when the day is hot or when you have to engage in physical activity. Drink before you even get thirsty. Drink plain, clean water. It doesn't matter if it is sparkling or still, piping hot or on the rocks. Have it with a drop of fresh lemon if it helps you drink enough.

Water activity is a scale to measure the amount of available water in food. Pure water has the water activity value of 1. Anything that is dissolved in water is called a solute. Solutes like sugar, salt, alcohol, and other nutrients added to water reduce the water activity.

This means that a food or beverage with more solute dissolved in it has less function as a source of water than pure water.

When choosing a thirst-quenching, body-fluid-replenishing

beverage, it is better to drink plain water or drinks with very few ingredients dissolved in them, such as lightly brewed unsweetened teas and some brands of diet beverages.

Juices, milk, sweetened drinks, soft drinks, energy drinks, alcoholic beverages, and soups don't count as good sources of water because of their high-solute content.

Fresh, plain water is ultimately the ideal source of water to stay hydrated.

Drink No Calories

There are two benefits to sticking with this rule:
1. You get more hydration from your beverage (as discussed in the previous section).
2. You avoid consumption of excess calories, which are more likely to be empty calories from refined carbohydrates.

This rule alone can help reduce most people's daily calorie intake by a quarter, if not more.

Most of us don't realize how many calories we consume when we drink juice, non-diet soft drinks, sweetened coffees and teas, lattes and other milk-based drinks. Not following this "Drink No Calories" rule often leads to the following:

- Overconsumption of sugar
- Overconsumption of calories
- Overeating caused by hunger swings, which are due to sugar consumption.

Foods in liquid form tend to go down the hatch quickly and mindlessly since there is no need to scoop, bite, and chew. When we drink our food, most of the time we're not even aware of the quantity we consume. Often we drink more of calorie-rich, sweetened beverage than we would water because the low-water activity of the beverage actually leaves us thirsty for more.

Drinking alcoholic beverages is best kept a recreational activity. Alcohol is intoxicating, and we all know the consequences of overindulgence. Treat it like chocolate; indulge in a little every once in a while, but don't make it a staple.

About 99 percent of the time, drink no calories.

Drinking no calories leaves us with limited choices on what we can drink most of the time:

- Water—still, sparkling, with a dash of lemon or herb
- Coffee and tea—black and unsweetened
- Diet soda

This is one of the easiest rules to stick to. It may also be, for some individuals, the most effective measure for quick calorie reduction and perhaps excess fat loss. *So let's drink water to health!*

"No disease that can be treated by diet should be treated with any means." Maimonides

The Micro-nutrients

- **Minerals**

Most of our dry body weight constitutes minerals. These minerals are deposited in bones. Bones provide the frame that protects the organs and supports muscles to enable mobility.

One thing we have to understand is that bones are dynamic. Minerals move into and out of bone tissue all the time. We need to replenish these minerals through proper nutrition—by consuming foods rich in calcium, phosphorous, and other salts for bone building.

Other minerals found in the body are dissolved in the body fluids. This process aids in biochemical reactions that are essential to life.

Salts like sodium, potassium, and chloride are involved in the electrical conduction in nerve and muscle cells.

Trace minerals like iodine, manganese, zinc, and selenium are essential for optimal biochemical processes.

Minerals are found in whole foods. A diet based on meat and vegetables is certain to be adequate in mineral content.

- **Vitamins**

Vitamins are essential in our diets because the human body cannot produce them. Vitamins are organic compounds that are necessary for biochemical reactions. Some of these vitamins, such as vitamins A, C, and E, are known for their protective antioxidant activity.

Vitamins are chemically and biochemically very diverse and can be separated into two broad categories—water soluble and fat soluble.

It is good to be mindful of this characteristic of vitamins if we want to be sure we get enough of them in our diets.

Water-soluble vitamins are vitamins C and the various vitamin Bs.

Oil-soluble vitamins are vitamins A, D, E, and K.

Literature on vitamins, minerals, and phytochemicals—as well as their sources and benefits—are available online and in books. There is generally no need for us to consume vitamin supplements. A diet that is complete with fish, meats, eggs, and fresh vegetables would contain sufficient amounts of micronutrients needed for a healthy existence.

Diet Myths of the Twenty-First Century

The last three decades have seen the largest increase in obesity rates among populations in the developed world. This is despite the fact that there is more awareness and more information about it.

Part of the problem is that the information given to us over the last decades was not completely accurate. Some of the worst advice we got are the myths, which many of today's writers of good books on nutrition and weight loss have tried to debunk.

The best way to discuss diet is to first focus on nutrition. Good nutrition comes only from a diet of good-quality food packed with the necessary macronutrients and micronutrients. Good-quality food keeps the body healthy. A healthy body can do wonders. It is full of energy; it can do things, replenish itself, and stay young.

The opposite is true for poor diets.

Eating poorly actually accelerates the aging process more quickly than lacking exercise.

Diet Myths to Debunk Forever

There are numerous diet myths that need to be debunked. These myths have misled us into decades of misinformation and the obesity epidemic. There are many theories as to how the myths have come to be so ingrained in our beliefs. Our concern here is to identify the most damaging of diet myths and debunk them.

Myth 1: Whole grains are healthy.
Truth: As mentioned earlier, whole grains are, like refined grains,

empty sources of carbohydrates. These cause insulin levels to rise just as badly as refined carbohydrates and starchy vegetables.

Myth 2: Fat in food causes obesity.
Truth: Uncontrolled carbohydrate consumption, not the fat in food, that leads to hunger swings causes overeating and obesity. Good fats in food have essential function, while refined carbohydrates only get stored up as fat.

Myth 3: A vegetarian diet is healthier.
Truth: A vegetarian diet gives no benefit because it is difficult to get adequate amounts of protein from vegetable sources. It is also difficult to get a good variety of food to ensure there is no deficiency in any nutrient.
Unless one is very well versed in vegetarian nutrition (or if one has motives other than health to go vegetarian), it is best not to adopt a strict vegetarian diet.

Myth 4: Egg yolks are bad because they contain cholesterol.
Truth: Egg yolks contain cholesterol, yes. Egg yolks are also a cheap source of vital nutrients. Furthermore, cholesterol is not a harmful substance. Cholesterol molecules are found in our cell membranes that keep cell structure flexible and functional. The body regulates its own production of cholesterol with cholesterol in the diet.

Myth 5: Cholesterol causes heart disease.
Truth: The cholesterol we're led to believe is the "bad cholesterol" that causes heart disease isn't even cholesterol. It is a large molecule called "type-B low-density lipoprotein" (LDL).
Type-B LDL levels in the blood are controlled by reducing visceral fat accumulation (fat around the waist) by embarking on a low, controlled carbohydrate diet and exercise.

If your meals are predominantly made up of refined carbohydrates and you find yourself needing a snack not two hours later, it's time to change the menu. We can see that the bulk of problems we face today are associated with diets consisting of predominantly refined carbohydrates. It is sensible to ignore myths and focus on eliminating the real dietary culprits.

The Dangers of Poor Diet

The human body is not formed as static material but is in constant flux. Cells continually get damaged due to age and wear, and need replacement. This regenerative process depends on an adequate supply of macronutrients and micronutrients derived from the food we eat.

Nutrients are the building blocks of cell growth. Excessive or long-term calorie-deficient and/or nutrient-deficient diets deprive the body of its ability to regenerate itself, leading to breakdowns in tissue integrity and organ function. This deterioration happens gradually. The symptoms would be chronic in nature and will show up as signs of aging; fatigue; poor mental state; bone, muscle, and organ degeneration; cardiovascular disease; and a compromised immune system leading to infectious ailments and even cancer due to a weak immune system.

Malnutrition is a detriment to health. The irony is that while we, people in this modern world, think we have too much to eat, the reality is that most of us don't get enough of the essential nutrients in our diets to maintain good form.

LONG-TERM CALORIE DEFICIENCY

Calorie-deficient diets include excessive fasting, skipping meals, eating less, constantly going hungry, excessive calorie counting, going on a perpetual low-calorie diet, and struggling with anorexia. Most people go on a calorie deficit with the aim of losing weight. The premise is that if you eat fewer calories than you burned, you will lose weight.

The energy deficit brings about loss in fat for only the first couple of weeks; then it stops. Some people even find themselves putting the pounds back on.

A long-term calorie deficit puts the body into a starvation mode. The resting metabolic rate (RMR) goes down to conserve energy for survival.

This is a natural survival mechanism of human physiology, meant to sustain us in time of famine, which in Paleolithic times didn't last too long.

In this mode, fat is spared, defeating the dieter's purpose for going on the diet in the first place. More threatening to health is that biological processes considered nonessential for immediate survival, such as cell rejuvenation, muscle growth, bone replacement, and neurological and immune function, will slow to a halt. When this happens, everything slowly breaks down. This is the precursor to aging and aging-related diseases. Hence this method of dieting is not the solution to getting forever young and fit.

NUTRITION DEFICIENCY

Nutrition-deficient diets come in many forms. They include low-fat or no-fat diets, low-carbohydrate diets, and vegetarian diets.

Deliberately denying the body of any nutrient is like taking away the building blocks for growth and replenishment. It is the surest way to kick-start deterioration of the organs and accelerate the aging process.

Fat, protein, and carbohydrates all have a role in protecting the body from aging and illness. Nutrient-deficient diets have no place in our aim to stay young and fit.

MINDLESS EATING

Eating anything on hand, with the tendency to consume calorie-dense processed food, may seem like the opposite of calorie- and nutrient-deficient diets, but there is a similarity—it's a cause of malnutrition. Processed food, fast food, junk food, and the like are calorie dense and nutrient empty. This means that a small quantity of food can easily make up one's daily calorie needs without fulfilling the nutrient needs.

The high calories consumed with this kind of diet come predominantly from refined carbohydrates. As explained in the section on insulin, excessive refined-carbohydrate intake will cause obesity and metabolic disorder, leading to chronic diseases. Contrary to popular understanding, being fat doesn't mean being well nourished. You can put on fat and still have a body starving for vital nutrients.

EMOTIONAL EATING

Foods with addictive ingredients, such as sugar, carbohydrates, and alcohol, have calming and pleasurable effects on us. When we consume food to justify a poor emotional state, we're participating in emotional eating. Like taking narcotics and depression drugs, eating to feel better has only a transient effect. Emotional eating often leads to gross overeating and obesity.

Stop emotional eating by being aware of it and getting the appropriate help in curing the poor emotional state.

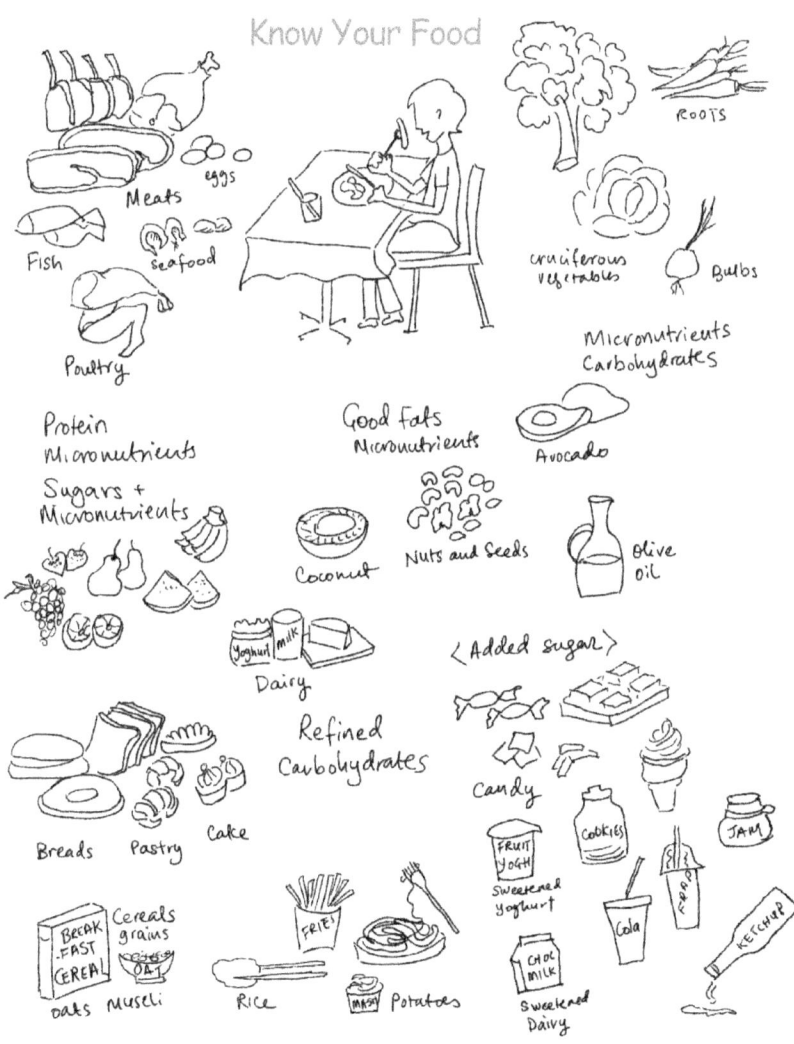

The Young-and-Fit Diet

Eat for replenishment and growth. Consider your nutrition mindfully. This is the philosophy for a diet practice that would keep you young and fit for life. A good attitude toward eating right has to do with the following attributes:

- **Mindfulness**

Be aware of everything you eat. Anything you put into your system during meals or outside of mealtime constitutes your diet. Being mindful helps us break nasty habits that add on empty calories. Habits include nibbling on snacks, tasting morsels of food offered at supermarkets, finishing up your kid's leftovers, eating free bread sticks at restaurants, and so forth.

- **The Macro-nutrient Shift**

Get enough protein and fat in your diet. These macro-nutrients should make the bulk of your daily meal. Plan your meals around protein-containing foods. Supplement your meals with good-quality dietary fats.

- **Selective Carbohydrate Sources**

Control your carbohydrates. These should come from non-starchy vegetables, nuts, and seeds. Avoid grains, starchy vegetables, and processed foods that contain sugar.

- **Quality of Choice**

Eat only quality food for micronutrients. The fresher the meats, fruits and vegetables, and so forth, the closer these foods are to their original state. Therefore, the more vitamins, phytochemicals, and minerals you will get from them.

- **Wholesomeness**

Choose whole foods over processed food. Processing depletes food of its natural micronutrients. Chemical additives added for the shelf-life extension of food need to be detoxified by the liver. This puts unnecessary stress on the organ.

- **Variety**

Eat a variety of food. This is a good habit to ensure you get all the nutrients the body needs. It is also a safeguard against accumulation of chemicals or an overdose of certain micronutrients in the body.

Eating to stay young and fit is only about getting the right amount of nutrients for the purpose of building and replenishing tissues and organs.

Forget Calorie Counting

"A good decision is based on knowledge and not on numbers."
Plato

A calorie is a unit measure of energy. The food "calories" we see on food labels are calculated in a physics laboratory by measuring the amount of heat emitted when a food sample is ignited in a bomb calorimeter. Corrections in the readings are sometimes made with consideration to the digestibility and absorption of particular food types in an attempt to reflect more closely the biological processing of the food.

The reality is different. The human body doesn't function like a bomb calorimeter. We don't combust our food. Different sets of enzymes in different tissues metabolize fats, proteins, and carbohydrates, and different hormonal mechanisms regulate them.

Our digestive system also absorbs different foods differently. Foods that are highly processed get digested, and their nutrients are absorbed into the blood more efficiently than whole, mildly cooked foods.

There are so many variables in the digestion, absorption, and metabolism of food that it is impossible for science to accurately calculate the "calories" in food products.

It is, therefore, better not to get number bound. Calories mean almost nothing in the reality of food and nutrition. We can use the calorie scale to estimate how much we eat. This estimation will not indicate whether the food we eat will keep us healthy or make us fat.

For example, calories from a piece of steak will have a different effect on your body than the same amount of calories from a pancake. The nutrients absorbed from the two sources of food will also have different functions.

Steak is protein rich and almost carbohydrate free. Consumption of steak releases amino acids in the blood. There will be an insignificant blood-sugar spike and very little insulin production.

A stack of pancakes, on the other hand, is carbohydrate rich. Eating pancakes will boost blood-sugar levels and lead to an insulin response.

This is an example of how two meals that measure the same number of calories in a calorimeter affect different hormonal responses. Depending on other dietary parameters and an individual's physical state, the rise in insulin levels from eating pancakes poses a greater potential for immediate fat storage than a similar calorie-containing meal of steak.

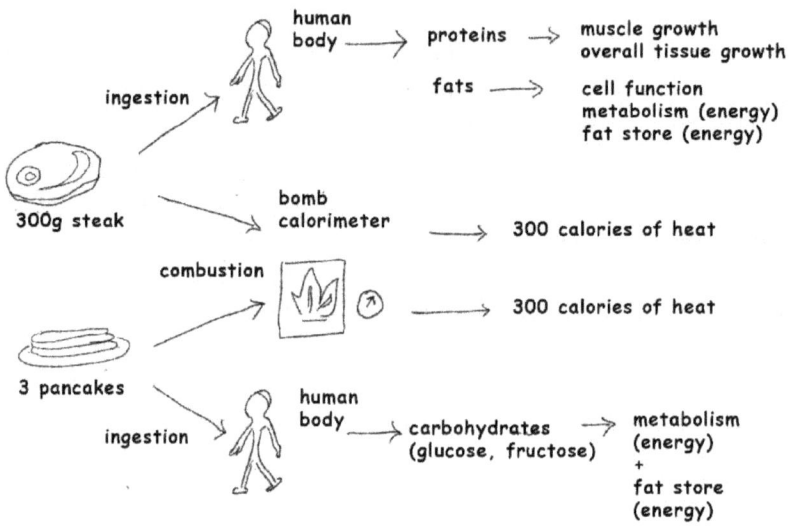

Both servings of meat and pancakes might burn in a caloriemeter to liberate 300 calories of energy, but in the human body, both are processed differently and used for different biochemical function.

Here is another example. Calories from apple juice will create a metabolic response in the body that is different from the same amount of calories from whole cut apple pieces. While the nutrients of both apple juice and whole apples are the same, the physical structures of the two foods are different. In whole fruit, nutrients are packed in cells and fiber, which hamper the digestion process of its nutrients.

The nutrients from whole apples get into the blood at a much lower rate and less efficient manner than apple juice because of the soluble and insoluble fibers still present in whole apples. Drinking apple juice causes a quick rise in blood glucose and fructose levels—hence a higher insulin response. Eating whole apple pieces results in a slower absorption of sugars into the bloodstream. This process gives more time for the sugars to be metabolized, requiring less insulin involvement.

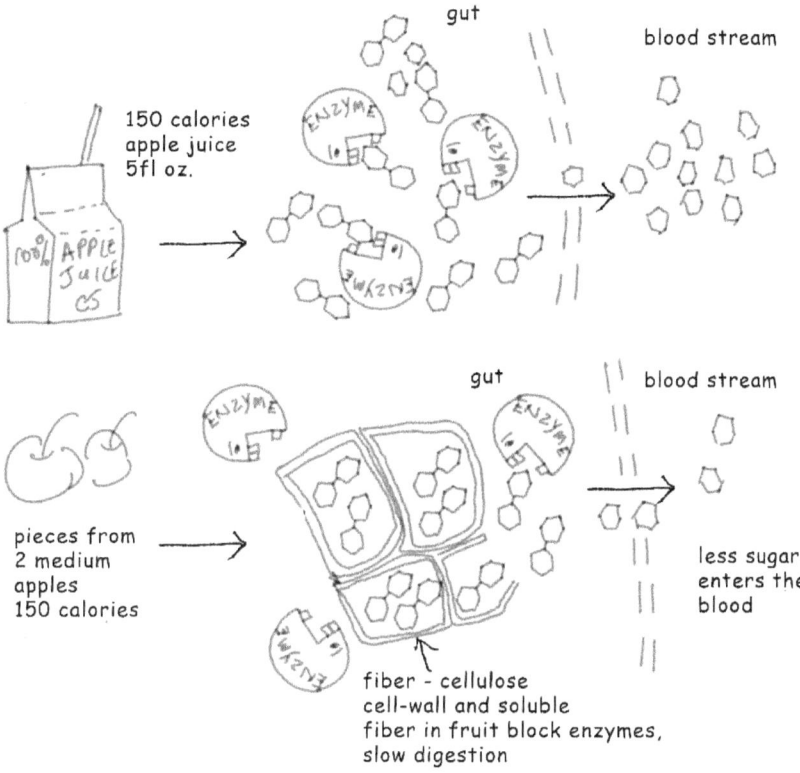

150 calories
apple juice
5fl oz.

gut

blood stream

pieces from
2 medium
apples
150 calories

gut

blood stream

less sugar
enters the
blood

fiber - cellulose
cell-wall and soluble
fiber in fruit block enzymes,
slow digestion

= sucrose (sugar molecule)   = glucose , fructose molecules

If knowing the number of calories doesn't help us stay healthy or lean, what is the point of counting calories in the first place? There isn't. As stated in the chapter on exercise, this is the same reason why we should not be too concerned about counting calories.

We don't get fat just because we eat too many calories. We accumulate fat in our bodies because we eat calories from the wrong *food source.*

The good news is that we don't need to eat less. We just need to eat differently. A diet consistently dominated by carbohydrates (especially refined carbohydrates) stimulates insulin production. The body becomes a fat-accumulating, fat-sparing, and carbohydrate-burning machine. This is the diet prevalent in almost every part of the developed world. This is the diet of today's obesity epidemic.

To solve these constant obesity concerns, immediately make these changes to the diet:

- Reduce the carbohydrates in your diet, while consuming more protein and fat.
- Replace all refined carbohydrates you normally consume at mealtime with fresh meat, fish, poultry, non-starchy vegetables, some fruit, legumes, nuts, seeds, mushrooms, and eggs.
- Avoid foods containing high quantities of fructose and alcohol. Enjoy these but only in homeopathic quantities.

A change in diet—to one that is very low in refined carbohydrates, sugars, and alcohol; and is rich in good-quality protein, fat, and fresh vegetables—will cause a good change in the metabolic machinery. With a low incidence of blood sugar surges leading to insulin spikes, fat burning will start to kick in. It may take a couple of weeks for this change to happen, but it will happen. When the cells in the body start to burn fat, fat loss becomes a long-term reality.

Healthiness and Not Thinness

There is no harm in having a little fat here and there or now and then. We need to focus on being healthy, not thin. Good health is possible only if your body is fed right. A healthy body is a young body.

The bonus is that eating right raises your metabolism and improves your energy levels. This will almost automatically work in your favor to reduce excess body fat.

Simple Meal Planning

Planning your meals is a good way to keep yourself on a clean diet. Meal planning isn't about making spreadsheet tables so you have to plan what you want to eat days in advance. That can be complicated and impossible to follow through on. It is more effective to take a look at every aspect of the meal—the where, when, and how—rather than to focus only on the what. Here are some ideas:

- Have meals only at the dining table, not in front of the television or at the work desk.
- Focus on what you eat while you eat. When you're aware of your eating, you're less likely to overeat. Refrain from eating on the move or in front of distraction like the television.
- Start every meal with the right kind of food. Fill your belly first with lean meats, eggs, and vegetables before going for anything else.
- Snack wisely. Nuts—especially raw, lightly roasted, and unsalted ones—are great. Fruit, vegetable sticks, boiled eggs, and some cheese can also make good snacks. Snacks being snacks, they should be eaten mindfully.
- Drink water before and after every meal to feel satiated more quickly.
- Eat slowly. About twenty minutes need to pass before your body realizes you have had enough.
- Learn to stop eating when you're not hungry anymore. This takes a little practice. Be conscious of the differences between feeling hungry, feeling not hungry anymore, feeling full, and feeling stuffed.
- Don't completely deprive yourself from the foods you love; however, reduce your exposure to them. Do enjoy them in small amounts, as a treat every once in a while.

Healthy Eating as a Lifestyle

"Going on a diet" is something you may do on the short term. Most diets are unsustainable. They are either too depressing to follow or unhealthy. True healthy eating for staying young and fit is a permanent lifestyle choice. That is why you shouldn't overanalyze, count, weigh, or make big diet charts.

All you have to do is understand that your reason for choosing what you eat is for the sole purpose of good body function, which is the prerequisite of staying young and fit. Experiment with different foods. Our bodies react differently to different eating patterns and habits. Understanding how your body works is the answer to managing your health.

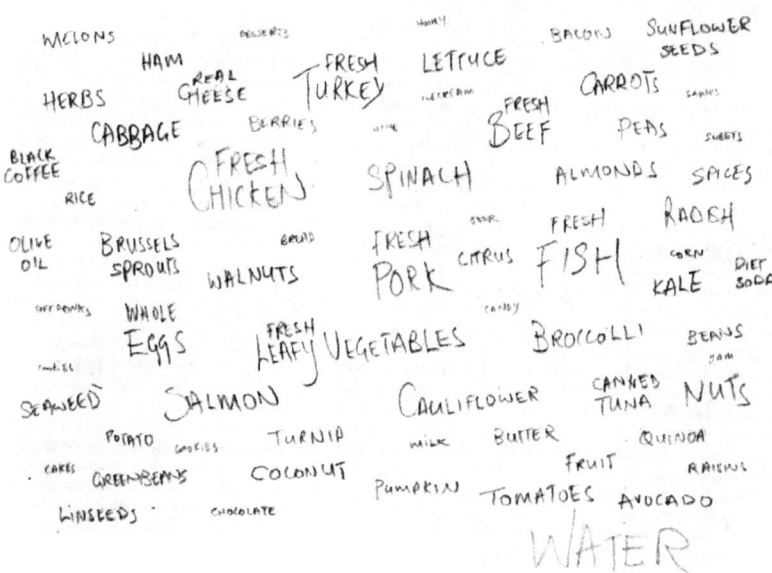

Smart Grocery Shopping

Not everybody enjoys grocery shopping, and the food industry is aware of that. If it is not entertaining or interesting, we don't buy. This is how companies are able to genetically select food crops, modify, package, and color lesser-quality food and get more sales.

It is time to change our attitudes toward grocery shopping. Imagine a woman from Paleolithic times going out into the wilderness to gather daily staples. How would she have done it? Would she have selected the brightest-colored thing just because it looked interesting? No, because brightly colored plants and grubs in nature are likely to be poisonous. The woman would have picked the freshest things available and only those she had learned from previous generations to be edible and nutritious.

Would a caveman pick up a dead animal rather than hunt for a live beast just because it was easier to get? I would think not, because he probably understood that rotten flesh can be deadly.

Modern society is in love with processed food. Instead of being more discerning, we have forgotten the importance of nutrition for survival. Thinking about food quality can be boring, so we allow ourselves to be manipulated. To sell more, food processors add color, shape, packaging, and all kinds of marketing slogans to entice us into picking out their produce at the grocery store.

When we thoughtlessly give convenience and packaging precedence over the nutritional quality of food, we choose wrong. When we choose wrong, we eat wrong.

Grocery Shopping Made Simple

A good way to get only quality nutrition through grocery shopping is to stock your cart with healthy items while leaving unhealthy food on the shelves. We can also follow this simple rule:

- Let 80 percent of food in your shopping cart contain raw, whole, unprocessed meats, fish, eggs, and non-starchy vegetables and fruit.
- Let 15 percent contain some cheese and delicatessen, nuts and seeds, butter, good oils, canned fish, coffee, and tea.
- Let 5 percent be anything else.

If you want to transform your life today, refrain from stocking up on foods that contain added sugar, refined carbohydrates, and alcohol. These are usually over-processed and ready to eat. Experience has shown that the more of these foods we keep at home, the more of them we consume.

Smart grocery shopping is the key to eating right at home.

Strategies for Dining Out

Eating establishments are in the business of making profits from the food they serve you. In order to achieve that, these businesses have to focus on everything else but serving healthy food. Some of the strategies restaurants use include the following:

- Stuffing the menu with cheap, refined carbohydrates so the dishes look bigger
- Over-seasoning, as in adding too much salt, MSG, and other artificial flavor ingredients to mask lesser-quality cooking or poorer-quality food
- Using trans fats for frying, because the oil can be re-used in the fryer much longer than healthier fats

- Deep-frying or frying everything with a lot of fat because it cooks the food more quickly
- Adding starch and sugar to food, especially sauces, gravies, and salad dressings for a more attractive look and taste
- Serving huge portions to look like more value for the money. This causes the consumer to overeat.

For most of us, dining out is no longer something we do only on special occasions. It has become a necessity. Some of us even dine out every day.

Apart from the obviously unhealthy fare, most restaurants also serve healthy alternatives. Many restaurants also take special requests from their customers. We, therefore, have a choice of choosing food that is right for us while dining out. All we need is a strategy:

Before Ordering Food

- If you know the restaurant menu already, plan in advance what you can eat there. If you don't know the restaurant or are unsure what is on the menu, try not to go there in a ravenous state. Have a small healthy snack beforehand.
- Your beverage order should ideally be limited to water, diet soda (if you have to), unsweetened tea, or coffee.
- Send back the free bread, chips, nuts, or whatever between-meal snack is provided.

What to Order

- Pick the dish with a larger serving of whole lean protein. It could be a whole chicken breast, a steak, fish, pork, beef, venison, lamb, or eggs.
- Get a good serving of vegetables. These should be mainly greens, cruciferous vegetables, stems and roots, non-starchy vegetables, and vegetables cooked as lightly as possible without too much sauce and seasoning. Salads and steamed vegetables are normally good choices.
- If the dish comes with a serving of fries, pasta, or rice, ask if you could substitute them with more vegetables.
- Ask for sauce on the side. Sauces and gravies normally contain sugar, starch, fat, and too much salt. Having them on the side allows you to control how much of that you eat. No ketchup please!

How to Eat

- Eat the meat and vegetables first before consuming the other components of the dish. Undigested proteins and fiber in the stomach tend to satisfy hunger quickly, making you less likely to binge on the carbohydrates.

- Eat slowly.
- Stop eating when you're no longer hungry.
- Drink water between mouthfuls.
- Leave as much of the potatoes, bread, pasta, and rice—the carbohydrate-rich foods—behind as possible. Remember that carbohydrates are cheap stuffing restaurants put on plate to give consumers the impression they are getting more value for their money. We know that consuming refined carbohydrates is the cause for a host of health issues. Understand that leaving them behind is not a waste. They are simply not worth eating.
- Skip dessert or—maybe, why not?—share your dessert.
- Have black coffee or tea without sugar.
- Eating out will not be a healthy-diet-busting activity. Plan ahead what you will and will not eat before entering a restaurant. If you're invited to a restaurant that doesn't offer healthy options in its menu, have a healthy snack beforehand so you don't go with an empty stomach.

Enjoy Your Special Occasions

Just because you're on the path of a healthy lifestyle doesn't mean you cannot enjoy fun foods on special occasions. It is good to forget restrictions every once in a while and give yourself a treat. Your body can take incidental onslaughts of naughty food.

If your lifestyle is generally about eating clean, you can afford to party. This is actually good for you. The process of staying forever young, forever fit is about replenishment. Enjoyment with friends and family over fun food sends pleasure hormones into your body. Your body will de-stress, and your immune system will get a boost, even if you have that champagne and four servings of chocolate cake.

MENU

Spaghetti Alfredo

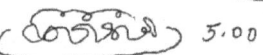

5.00

> Dish dominated by carbohydrate is not a good choice

BBQ Chicken Tighs
with Fettuccini Pasta

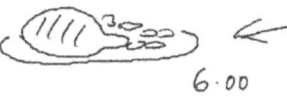

6.00

> Choose instead the dish with larger serving of lean protein.

MENU

Chicken Cordon Bleu
with Fries

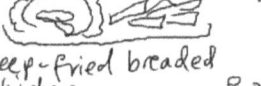

Deep-fried breaded
chicken   8.00

> Deep-fried meat is not a good choice.

Pork Chops with
Fries

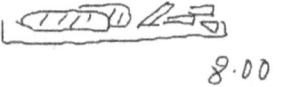

8.00

> Better to have meat that is not deep-fried but grilled.
> Do ask for vegetables instead of French-fries, or leave the fries un-eaten.

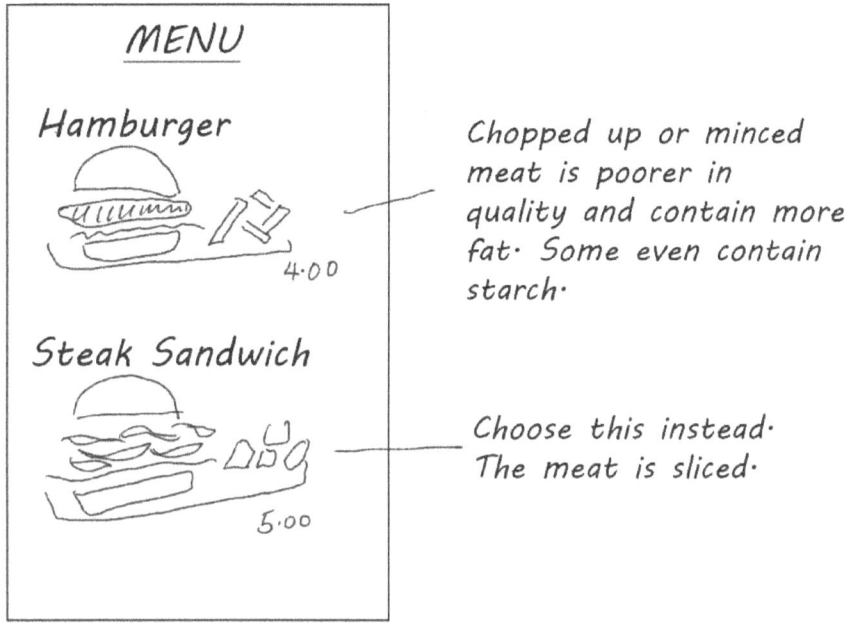

MENU

Hamburger

4.00

Chopped up or minced meat is poorer in quality and contain more fat. Some even contain starch.

Steak Sandwich

5.00

Choose this instead. The meat is sliced.

Diet is a Big Part of Staying Young and Fit

This is a big chapter because nutrition affects the state of our health more than anything else, even physical exercise. Everything you eat affects your physiology sooner or later.

Eat well to live well. Eat mindfully with the aim of getting the essential macronutrients and micronutrients.

Understand your own body. Try different foods and observe the effect food has on your health. You will see a great transformation in your physical form by adjusting your diet in the right direction.

Once you've got the hang of eating well, grocery shopping, cooking, and dining out will be a pleasure. There will be no confusion, doubts, or the feeling of overeating—or the idea that you need to abstain from anything enjoyable.

Maintaining healthy eating habits is a lifestyle anyone can adopt by following certain rules. Adhere to these rules as closely as possible. They do get easier with perseverance. There are many ways to motivate ourselves to eat well. For some of us, the obvious positive effects of our clean diet are motivation enough. There are also books to read on proper nutrition, and even self-hypnosis recordings that can sort out any cause for eating poorly.

Do whatever it takes to keep on track. Try to understand what works for you to stay forever young and fit.

Chapter 6: Build, Don't Burn

Being forever young and fit is a mission built on many tiny goals we set for ourselves. Only goals that are based on solid ideas will leave long-lasting impact. In this chapter we discuss the fundamental principles behind this lifestyle makeover.

"Build, don't burn" is the foundation on which these goals are built. Get this right by choosing foods and an exercise regime with the goal of building, and every effort put in will bring success. Get it wrong, and efforts will bring only diminishing returns.

This reinforcement of the previous chapters carries with it the most important message in this book. This message sets this book apart from many weight-loss and diet programs. These programs tend to harp on fat loss, calorie burning, and weight loss—everything done to "lose" something.

Losing fat is not like going into a cupboard full of groceries and taking only the butter out. When we diet and exercise just to burn fat without any consideration for building and regenerating, we burn everything else together with the fat. "Everything else" includes useful tissues such as muscles, skin, the brain, the immune system, and so forth.

Loss leads to deterioration. Deterioration leads to poor health and aging.

A sensible program works toward building the body to become a healthy machine for using fat as a fuel. Reduction in adiposity is a healthy consequence of being young and fit, not the means. This is what "build, don't burn" is all about.

Aging is Beyond Skin Deep

Erasing wrinkles, plumping up sagging skin, hiding gray hairs, and losing weight are examples of superficial ways to look younger. Those with the means can achieve "results" with one trip to the cosmetic surgeon's office. Removing the signs of aging in this way does nothing to remove the actual causes of aging.

We age from the inside out. Our physical appearance is a reflection of our state of health. Those who live in high mental and/or physical stress environments and individuals who lead an unhealthy lifestyle tend to look older than peers who take better care of themselves. Their prematurely aged appearance is a marker of a deteriorating state of health.

Deterioration happens very gradually. It is a process in which the entire person goes through physical, mental, and emotional losses. Observable physical deterioration includes the following:

- Loss of muscle mass, tone, and flexibility
- Loss of bone density
- Loss of skin integrity
- Loss of hormonal function (growth and reproductive function)
- Loss of neurological function
- Loss of organ functionality
- Mental deterioration such as loss of memory, loss of motor functions, and mental illness is the product of physical losses.

Emotional deterioration such as depression, loss of drive, loss of will, and so forth is the product of physical disability and mental losses. Emotional problems often lead to more physical deterioration. This then becomes a vicious cycle.

Loss is aging. To stop aging, we must stop the deterioration of our physical, mental, and emotional selves.

The first chapters of this book explained aging as the gradual process of deterioration and loss of physiological function. Since this is the case for all of us, getting *Forever Young, Forever Fit* is solely about achieving the opposite.

We're talking about building, maintaining, replenishing, and regenerating. Anything we do that doesn't build, replenish, or regenerate will not help our cause. Getting the right mind-set in our approach toward diet and exercise is essential.

Eat to Build

Eating is about nourishing the body so it can keep regenerating itself. Living tissues that make up our organs need nutrients to keep alive and flourish. When we talk about diet, our foremost concern is what we have to eat. We have to eat mindfully with the intent of getting enough macronutrients and micronutrients into our system.

The obesity crisis in today's world has caused us to believe that food is the enemy. That is wrong. Remember what we discussed in the last chapter, good food is your friend.

Too Much On Just Losing Weight Will Lead To Aging

If we want to fight aging and stay young, focusing on losing weight alone will cause us to achieve the opposite. Sacrifices that you put into dieting in this way will bring diminishing returns in the long haul. Conventional diets for losing weight commonly include one or more of the following regiments:

- Calorie deficiency (eat less)
- Fat deficiency (low-fat diet)
- Protein deficiency (very strict vegetarian diets)

The principle behind these diets is to consume fewer calories and/or fat than we need in an effort to "burn fat." The benchmark for progress is often measured by the numbers on the bathroom scale. If we lose some pounds on these kinds of diets, we think we're successful.

But what do we really want to achieve? Are we going to concern ourselves with a number on the scale at the expense of everything else? We should not do that because the numbers make only little sense. What we really want to achieve is not weight loss but excess fat loss.

What happens when we narrowly focus on "fat burning" during exercise or through dieting is lean body mass loss while fat loss is only temporary.

Lean-body mass loss means deterioration of muscles and other organs in the body. While we try to "burn calories" by consuming less food or doing more exercise, the body will draw its deficit energy from storage. This storage, we often hope, will come only from the fat cells in the adipose tissues—the cells that lie under the skin and cause us to look flabby. The problem is that this burning process isn't that precise.

Depending on what kind of weight-loss regime we put ourselves on, the body may burn fat along with proteins from muscles, skin, blood, and other organs. Getting thinner in this way leads to the deterioration of organs, which ages the body.

This is the reason why we often observe that

- individuals who go on extreme diets for long periods of time may be thin, but they look haggard and seem to age faster;

- individuals who do extreme cardio exercises for many years may have low body fat, but they also look drained, develop joint problems, and seem to age more quickly; and
- individuals who are thin don't necessarily live longer or healthier.

The sad truth about long-term deficient diets is that these fat-loss effects don't last. The body reacts to the lack of energy input and excess energy consumption by going on starvation mode. The RMR will decrease, while fat will be spared, stored, and locked up. When the dieter starts eating "normally" again, the fat piles back on with a vengeance, leading to the impulse to go on another diet. This is an example of a yo-yo diet phenomenon we know so well.

As explained in the last chapter, eating the right foods—in other words, whole foods that are rich in micronutrients and macronutrients, with low or no refined carbohydrates and sugar, is the only way to lose the excess body fat. Take simple carbohydrates and sugar out of your diet, and your hormonal profile will change. The body will gradually adjust to choosing fat over glucose as the main fuel of choice.

The good news is that eating to build means freedom from calorie counting and starving. It works synergistically with the right exercise regime and makes you lean in the long term. It is about ensuring that every meal you have is rich in nutrients that will feed the tissues in your body so the organs stay rejuvenated and in full function. It also makes your exercise more effective by allowing your muscles to grow with the effect of natural growth hormones.

A body that is well fed cannot go through the devastation of aging through deterioration. It will, in fact, be stored up with a lot of dynamic energy. Not the latent energy stored in fat cells but the energy that comes from strength of healthy cells in the organs, bones, skin, brain, and immune system.

Eating to build is eating to live, thrive and be forever young, forever fit.

Exercise to Build Muscle

When we discuss exercise, we focus on building muscles. We will not think about burning calories or fat. Workouts with focus on burning fats alone include long bouts of cardio—constant-paced long-distance running, hours of biking, or working out at the elliptical trainers, treadmills, and stair-climbing machines. These exercises (and the numbers on exercise machines) give the false impression that the longer we exercise, the more fat we will burn.

The more prolonged the exercise, more precious muscle, skin, and other tissues will be burned along with the fat. These kinds of exercises also set the body into starvation mode and a lowered RMR, so we use less energy at rest.

The body gets used to the cardio exercises within months, rendering them less effective for fat loss. When the exerciser does less, the fat piles back on again. Like the effect of the yo-yo dieter, the cardio exerciser just needs to spend more time exercising—a vicious cycle ensues.

When we exercise to build muscles, we grow new muscle tissue. The cells that make up the muscle tissue do the job of fat burning for us during and after a workout. The short duration of strength-training workouts reduces the risk of compromising other body parts along with burning fats.

Having more muscles means increased RMR. This means a higher metabolism rate at rest. The body consumes more energy just doing day-to-day activities. This in turn leads to an overall leaner, toned physique.

When we work to build muscles, our workouts will be different. Exercises to build muscle are so effective that we don't need to spend a lot of time working out.

Building muscles also means building strength. Strength leads to greater mobility as well.

Exercise to Build Bone

Bones are made of living, dynamic material. They are not like dead wood, which is static. Every day, new bone material is formed and reformed. This is how fractured bones heal.

The detriment of the aging process is loss of bone mass. It is a condition called osteoporosis. This disease can be prevented if we consciously seek to keep building our body by eating to build and exercising to build.

There is a mind-body connection. When you exercise to gain strength, after exercise your brain gets the message to build strength.

To get the strength, your muscles are told to grow. For your muscles to find support, your bones are told to regenerate. You eat well so that all the nutrients needed to build bone are available for the building and regenerative process.

This building and regenerative process takes place at a special time. It happens when you sleep.

Exercise to Build Nerve Fibers

Older people are known to suffer falls more frequently than younger people. This is because aging leads to gradual loss of nerve cells that connect the brain to muscles. Nerve fibers are the communication conduits between and brain and muscles. Deterioration of nerve cells leads to a slowdown in our ability to react when we lose our balance or trip over something. We suffer slower reaction time because there are fewer connections left between brain and muscles.

That is why true fitness includes balance. Exercises like yoga improve balance, stimulate nerves to regenerate, and keep us in proper balance for life.

The Importance of Sleep

Sleep is of paramount importance to health. It is absolutely necessary for building, maintaining, replenishing, and regenerating all physiological functions in our bodies. Sleep is necessary for life.

Sleep is an integral part of our biology. Human beings have evolved to sleep at certain hours of the day. This is somewhere between dusk and dawn, with the duration of about eight hours. It is part of our evolved circadian rhythm. Our hormones synchronize with the twenty-four-hour day-night cycle so we naturally feel like sleeping when the lights are out. When our clocks are set, they normally take a week to reset. We can feel helpless going against our clacks when we fly across continents and feel the effects of jet lag.

Sleep is the body's way of shutting down conscious and motor activity so precious energy can be channeled into rebuilding. This whole process involves a shift in hormonal activity that takes place as we sleep.

Hormones that help us move around, eat, and process our food—

everything we do while awake—make way for a new set of hormones.

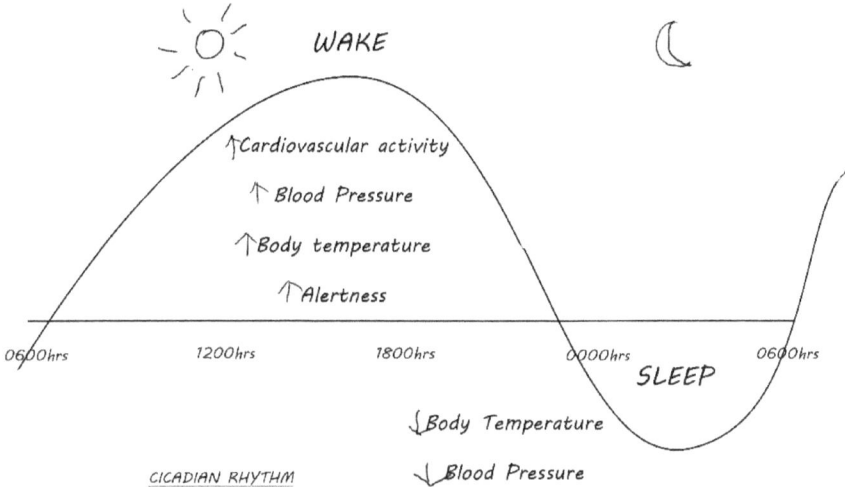

These hormones active at sleep, while shutting off physical activity, act to facilitate chains of biochemical reactions to rebuild, rejuvenate, and reset the body.

Wait. That sounds like the work of human growth hormones, doesn't it?

Yes. Human growth hormones, together with other synergistic hormones, are produced and take effect during sleep. The bonus of sleep is that it also helps us lose excess fat.

Late nights at work, in front of the TV or computer screen, at the bar, or doing any activity deprive the body of sleep. The overachievers' lifestyle of working hard and playing hard way into the wee hours of the morning achieves nothing more than the following:

- Gradual tissue deterioration, leading to organ dysfunction, loss in bone mass, skin damage, and muscle weakness
- Impairment of the immune system, leading to susceptibility to infectious diseases and cancer
- Metabolic disorders leading to obesity
- Accelerated aging

That is what we don't want.

Sleep. Don't just take a nap. Sleep deep.

The process of human sleep is cyclical and happens in stages. We go through four to five cycles of sleep on a good night. To get adequate sleep, we need to do the following:

- Sleep at night.
- Set yourself eight hours sleep. Go to bed at the appropriate time.
- Keep the room dark.
- Keep the room cool enough that you feel comfortable under blankets.
- Shut of all electronics, including any gadgets that could potentially set off alarms or alerts.

Watching TV, roaming the Internet, eating, and working in bed are habits that will rob bedtime sleep of time. If you save the bed only for sleep, your senses will associate relaxation with the touch of the sheets.

To completely unwind, close your eyes and breathe slowly. Focus only on that breathing.

It is true that each individual has a different need for sleep. However, this difference isn't really that great. The requirement still hovers around eight hours per night. Our sleep requirements can change over time. The amount of sleep we need depends on a whole load of factors—when we exercise more, for example. We might need to sleep longer.

Listen to your body and sleep whenever you can. The only way to realize your need for sleep is to stay away from stimulants. These stimulants may be artificial or otherwise, food related or activity related.

A change in attitude toward sleep might mean less time for partying or grinding at your work. But this change is worth it. Try sleeping more for a couple of weeks. You will notice a change in your body. You will lose weight, feel more energetic, and get less hungry. The most obvious change you may find with improved sleep is clearer skin. That is a marker for your overall improved health.

The Dangers of Stress

Stress has a counter-effect on the body and is just the opposite of sleep as far as its benefits. Situations that cause us stress stimulate a chain of events in the brain that lead to the secretion of stress hormones into the bloodstream. Stress hormones—in particular, cortisol—set into action chains of physiological responses to cope with the perceived stress situation.

The function of a stress response is to focus all energy in the body toward fight and flight. In a state of stress, energy gets drained from the organs. Cell-building activity is put on hold, and the body turns into an energy-burning machine. We feel it in our increased heart rate, blood pressure, and single-minded focus. Over time, people under stress either lose weight because of the energy drain or gain weight because the energy loss stimulates appetite. Losing or gaining weight due to stress can lead to long-term chronic ailments.

While sleep hormones act to rejuvenate the body, stress hormones act to shut down all rebuilding activity so the body can focus on tasks to overcome stressful situations.

Stress is useful for survival only if we really need to get away from dangerous situations. These situations rarely ever happen; and if they do, they last only short spurts of time.

If we allow daily activity to stress us out, we expose our body to those organ-burning hormones all the time. Continual exposure to stress hormones leads to loss of vital regenerative functions. This leads to aging. In severe situations, the effect of stress is manifested in chronic diseases like hypertension, cardiac disease, dementia, cancer, and other degenerative diseases.

Learn to Relax

Even though there are infinite causes of stress, it is safe to generalize that stress happens as a result of holding on to expectations.
Expectations are needs. Unmet needs become disappointments. Some of these are neurotic needs, which are actually crazy ideas and limiting beliefs. Those kinds of needs are like bottomless pits.

We suffer stress because we don't let go of our expectations. Stress isn't worth the loss of good health. Let go of stress by letting go of the needs.

When a situation engulfs us, our vision gets clouded. The mind initiates stress responses in the body by interpreting environmental situations according to our individual needs. That is why different people faced with the same experience cope differently. It is about having a different perspective of the same thing.

Sometimes we need to sit back, step out of everything, and observe our lives from a distance. We often can see things differently when we change our point of view. We can reframe the situation and look at it from a new perspective.

A therapist can be of brilliant help with this to those who can afford to engage one. We can also help ourselves out of stressful situations by reading inspirational books and practicing regular meditation and self-hypnosis. The best way to get help is to ask people around you for help.

Reading inspiring books can help us reframe our thoughts and view our world through different lenses. Having a refreshed perspective of life through reading helpful books helps us heal our bodies from stress.

Each of us has a different life situation. We suffer stress. It is important to be conscious of the fact that eliminating stress is important for long-term health.

We need to learn to let go of expectations or any need that harms us by causing stress. There are many ways to go about this. We can talk to others, hire therapists, and take on activities that help us relieve stress such as dancing or playing the piano.

We can also learn to meditate, which is a powerful way to relax.

Meditation & Hypnosis for Relaxation

Meditation and self-hypnosis are powerful tools for relaxation.

Both produce states of deep relaxation by stilling parts of the body. Relaxation of the muscles frees up the mind. This is not unlike simulating paralysis of the body during sleep. During the process of meditation and hypnosis, however, the subject is really fully awake.

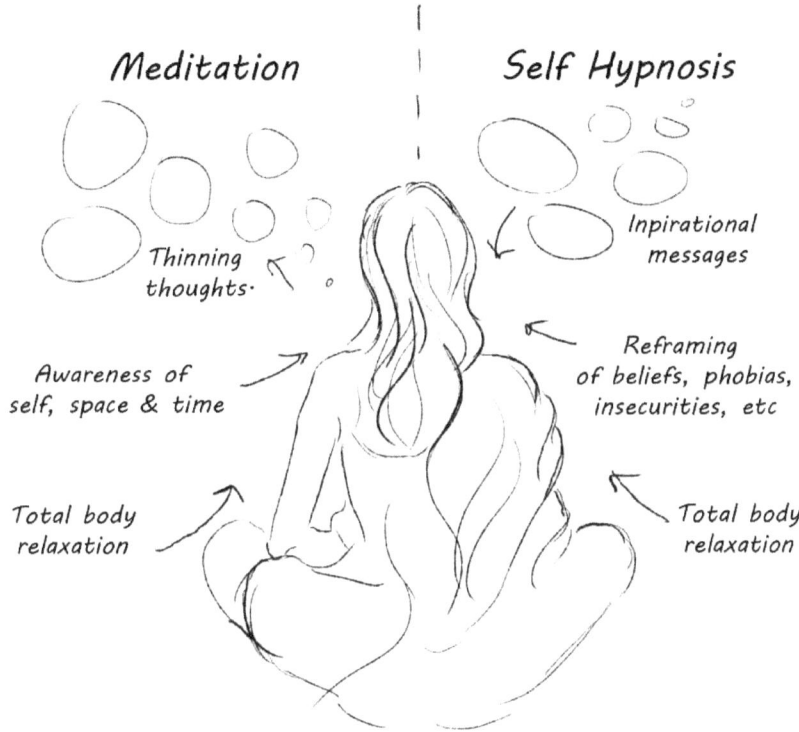

Meditation — Self Hypnosis

Thinning thoughts.

Awareness of self, space & time

Total body relaxation

Inpirational messages

Reframing of beliefs, phobias, insecurities, etc

Total body relaxation

MEDITATION

Meditation involves first emptying the mind of thought. It is not so easy for beginners to really do this. We think of our thoughts as conscious activity, but when we really try to rid our minds of thoughts, all manner of ideas pop into our heads. The ability to clear the mind of thoughts takes practice. It is possible for anyone to achieve this.

Mantras (or chants) and sounds can be played in the background during meditation to help the mind focus on something in the present. These are, however, unnecessary since some people meditate well in silence.

Find a safe and quiet place where you won't be disturbed for a couple of minutes. Sit or lie down in a comfortable posture. Close your eyes. Breathe naturally in smooth, continuous breaths. Focus on your breathing for a while, then very slowly scan every part of your body, relaxing the muscles as you go.

Pay attention to the relaxation of every single part of the body—the tips of the fingers and toes to the head. Remember to relax the shoulders, the facial muscles, and the tongue. Keep breathing naturally.

As the body relaxes, thoughts thin out, and the conscious mind goes into snooze, allowing the subconscious mind to open up to a different state of awareness.

Meditation is putting the body to sleep while waking up the mind. Your body goes into regenerative mode. You start building not only physical strength through relaxation but also emotional strength through heightened awareness.

SELF-HYPNOSIS

Self-hypnosis is a form of guided relaxation. It is also useful as therapy for emotional setbacks, insecurities, and phobias.

Unless one is experienced in this practice, the most effective method of self-hypnosis is relaxing while listening to a prepared hypnosis recording.

There are many sources of hypnosis recordings available for purchase or download from the Internet.

The preparation for self-hypnosis is similar to that of meditation—being in a comfortable posture, relaxing the muscles in the body, and breathing smoothly.

There is a structure to self-hypnosis. For the novice, the use of a self-hypnosis recording can be useful. These recordings are available as tapes or audio download. They are usually fifteen to forty minutes long and start with an induction to relax. This relaxation process is important because it helps open up the subconscious to the message. During relaxation, you're fully awake, focused on the message yet fully relaxed in the body. This is followed by the content. The content is the subject of the hypnosis session. There are numerous self-hypnosis recordings available in the market. For example, if you feel you need to overcome shyness and social anxiety, there is probably such a download with the message to help. The final part of the self-hypnosis session is the "waking up." Actually, you should be awake throughout the session, but this part is the ending, which helps you get back to reality.

One can do self-hypnosis without recordings. It is, however, a challenge for a novice to think of what to visualize. It is like trying to cut one's own hair.

Some sections of this book mention meditation or visualization. These are, in effect, methods of self-hypnosis.

What is self-hypnosis good for?

We all have thoughts, needs, limiting beliefs, and phobias that cause stress. These manifest in our lives as insecurities, anger, perfectionism, competitiveness, envy, and all manner of psychological encumbrances. Even if we're aware that these emotions are unwarranted, that they're all in our minds, we may be unable to shake them out of our heads.

This is because our emotional responses to real-life situations are hot-wired in our subconscious minds. Self-hypnosis gets to the subconscious part of the brain, unlocking these trapped, crazy ideas and freeing us from their hold on our feelings. This is an effective way to let go of stress. Having the mind focus on a message or visualization while in a relaxed state is like pressing a reset button. In doing so, we're better able to reframe our thoughts from negative to positive.

Stress, which the mind initiates, can be eliminated by changing the way the mind perceives situations. Meditation helps to clear the mind, bringing to focus the awareness of reality, while self-hypnosis resets beliefs through messages and visualization. Both practices work on the subconscious mind. They are powerful means of stress relief.

One can learn a lot of different methods of meditation and self-hypnosis. Like everything else, there is no single technique that works for everybody. The most successful people manage by exploring different ideas and learning what would suit them best.

Think "Build"

The mind and body are inextricably linked. This union holds a vast source of energy. This energy is like a battery that needs to be recharged. In their quest for success, in their striving to live life to the fullest, in their aim to stay healthy, many people forget that the body needs to regenerate, rejuvenate, and reset.

This is an important philosophy of an anti-aging lifestyle. Do nothing to cause your body to burn-out, like excessive low-calorie dieting or excessive cardio exercise. If you set fire to something, something else might burn along with it. That's how you stay young and fit—only through mind and body preservation.

Build Mentality	Burn Mentality
Exercise for fitness. Exercise to build muscle mass.	Exercise to burn calories Exercise to burn fat.
Diet based on getting adequate nutrients for growth.	Low calorie diet, low fat diet, restrictive diets.
Sleep.	Stress.
Meditation for relaxation	Stimulants, narcotics, smoking food and alcohol abuse.
Mindfulness	Neurosis

Chapter 7: What You See is What You Get

How do you really look? It's a funny thing. You're the only person in the world who cannot really see yourself in the flesh. Yes, you can see your hands, feet, belly, and some parts of your back, but you really cannot directly see your entire self. You cannot see how your body actually moves in space. We cannot even hear your real voice. Until we can peel our eyes out of our heads, and look at ourselves from afar, we wouldn't know how we really look. Photographs and videos give us some idea, but those images of us are not 100 percent realistic. Even if photography of a person were possible in 3-D, there would still be something missing.

When we look at ourselves in the mirror, that image is laterally inverted. Even if the mirror ran a mile long, we couldn't really see ourselves walk, run, sit, and stand naturally.

We cannot see ourselves, but the whole world can see us. From how we look, others make up their minds as to how young or old we are. Being forever young and forever fit is achieved when the world can see how young we *really* are. It would be pointless to let ourselves get old looking, frail, bent, or slouchy—and then try to tell the world, "I might look old, but I feel young."

Therefore, we need to be extra conscious of our looks.

There are many ways to go about analyzing your look. Videos can help with identifying and correcting posture issues. It would be a good idea to have someone take videos of how you walk, sit, and run, so bad posture habits can be noted and corrected.

Good posture is necessary for having that fit, youthful look. We shall discuss other features that give the impression of youth or youth long gone.

Some people neglect their looks for years, only to gasp, "OMG! Who is that old person wearing my dress in that video?"

That's the kind of surprise we want to do without. Instead, we want to surprise others by saying, "I will be one hundred tomorrow."

Look young to be young.

There are effective methods to achieving anything you want; you start from the outside in. You don't need to *be* young to *look* young. You look young to *be* young. This is not unlike the idea behind the saying "Fake it to make it." In this situation, I recommend the saying "Fake it to become it."

Counterintuitive? Perhaps it is. But it works. So why not try?

Let's assess what looking forever young, forever fit means. A couple of external factors affect how young we look. These are superficial markings of a young (or old) person. Let's work from the outside in.

Gait, Stride and Posture

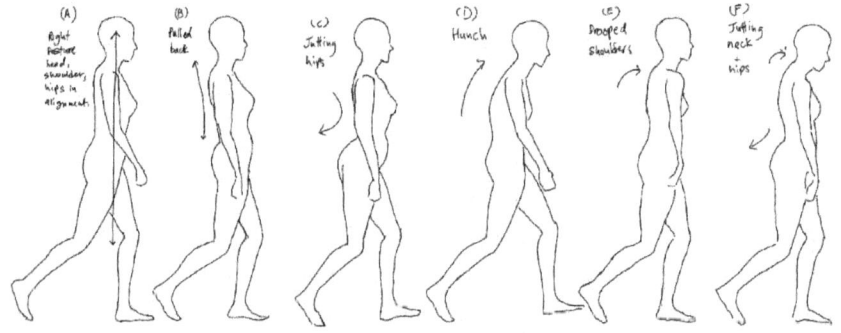

You can almost judge the health of a person by the way he or she moves. Exercise will help in this area. Better fitness brings better posture. Good posture brings the look of youthfulness. It is the first thing anyone will notice about you when you walk into a room.

You can also take extra care to move right. It is no effort if it becomes a habit.

Take a video of yourself walking as you normally walk. Look at the position of your head. Is the center of your head aligned with your shoulders? Or does your head jut forward or backward as you walk?

The best way to work on your walk is to exercise and to walk with the awareness of how you should walk. We might like to start doing the following easy things:

- Get good walking shoes.
- Walk on hills.
- Walk on uneven ground.
- Walk barefoot (but make sure the surface is free of sharp objects).

Always remember to align your head, shoulders, and hips and lift your feet.

The Skin Facts

One would expect a book like this to have a huge section on skin care loaded with advice on special cosmetic products, potions, and even plastic surgery.

The best strategy for staying young and fit is to do everything as naturally and simply as possible. This is the healthiest and least-risky way, and it can save you a lot of money.

Your skin is a very important organ in your body. The surface of the skin is what others see when they look at you. Since it covers the entire area of your body, it is also the organ most susceptible to damage.

It is the cumulative effect of damage that over time results in wrinkling, sagging, thinning, pigmentation and scars—the symptoms of aging skin.

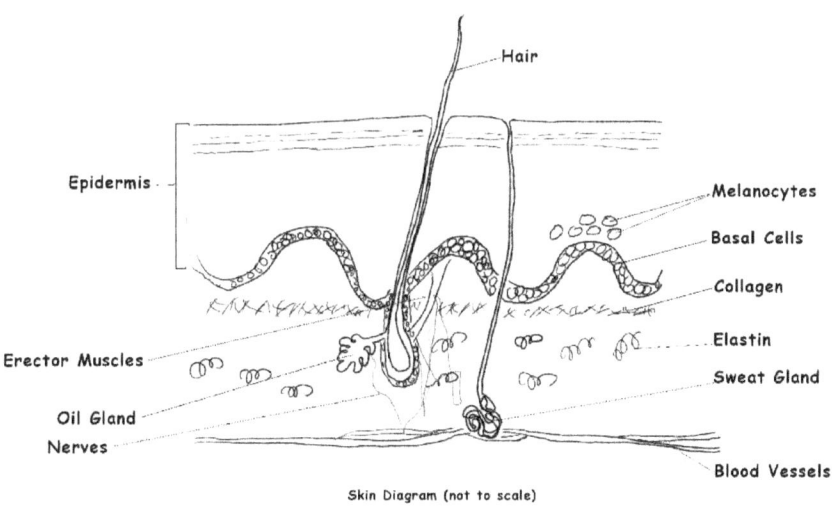

Skin Diagram (not to scale)

Damage the skin endures during a person's lifetime includes:
- Physical damage caused by cuts, scrapes, trauma, burns, and bites
- Chemical damage caused by contact with corrosive chemicals

- Radiation damage caused by overexposure to UV rays
- Allergy damage caused by the body's immune response to allergens
- Damage from the ingestion of contaminants due to smoking, ingesting alcohol, consuming sugar, and taking drugs
- Degeneration caused by poor nutrition and health
- Damage caused by illness and infections

Protection is the Best Form of Anti-Aging Skin Care

Skin regenerates itself constantly. Cells from the basal layer push upward and slowly dry up and drop off at the surface. Regeneration is necessary to retain the integrity of the skin as a barrier to protect the body from the external environment.

The best measure to keep skin from losing its integrity is to keep the degenerative processes at bay and protect skin from damage.

Creams, lotions, and cosmetic surgery are superficial measures to keep skin looking good, but they are no remedy for skin deterioration.

Skin, like every tissue in our bodies, must be built from the inside out. Skin cells need nutrients and stimulus to regenerate. The only way to provide these cells with food is via the bloodstream through good nutrition. Cells cannot receive food from outside the body.

The regeneration process keeps skin new, healthy, and looking young. New cells and protein structures like collagen and elastin are constantly formed to replace the old and damaged material. Hormones, like growth hormones, activate skin regeneration. This process requires energy and nutrients, which are fed to the skin. These nutrients can be obtained only via blood.

Help the skin's regeneration process by

- eating well so there is an adequate amount of nutrients feeding the skin;
- exercising to keep growth hormone levels up;
- preventing damage. Even though skin can replace itself, the process takes time. If damage overwhelms the healing process, scarring and permanent damage will occur.

Never a Safe Tan

Ultraviolet (UV) radiation from the sun carries with it energy that has the potency to cause destruction to molecules that make up the skin. When these molecules (like protein, fat, and DNA) are destroyed, skin structure gets damaged and loses its protective function.

A tan comes from skin defending itself from radiation. Cells called melanocytes produce a pigment, melanin, to absorb the sun's radiation in an effort to prevent more damage to other skin structures.

The skin's natural defense against radiation is limited. When it gets overwhelmed, protein molecules that make up structures like collagen and elastin start to break down. Actively duplicating melanocytes, the melanin-producing cells, also get damaged; these can mutate into cancerous forms.

Of all the possible damage one can do to one's own skin, radiation exposure is the most dangerous and should be avoided. Sadly, it is also the damage that is most self-inflicted.

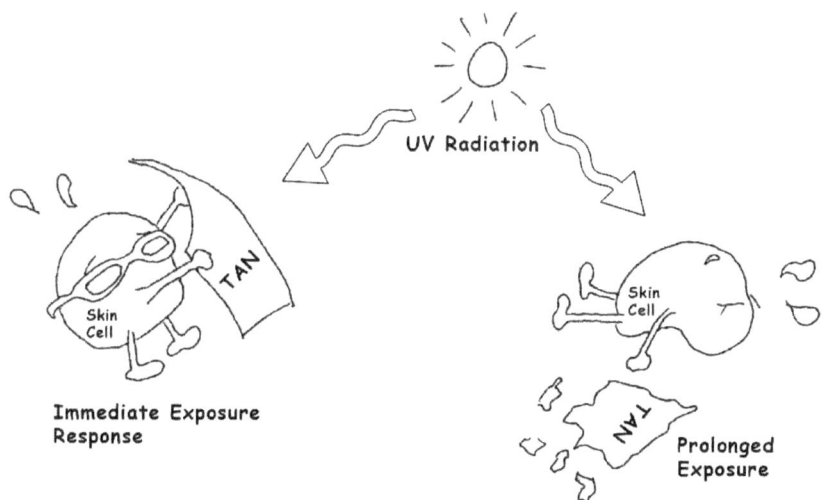

Avoid long exposure to the sun. Lying in the sun for hours—or worse, lying in a tanning bed, regardless of the type of "sun block" protection used—is dangerous to your skin.

Direct sunlight irradiates your skin with ultraviolet, UV, rays. These rays have enough energy to penetrate layers of skin cells. The energy affects the cells by attacking cell proteins and DNA. This

causes
- cell death, whereby the structure of the skin gets damaged; and
- cell mutation, which marks the beginning of cancer formation.

Sun exposure is necessary but only in regulated amounts. We need to spend only a few minutes each day enjoying the warmth of the sun. Sunlight is an excellent source of vitamin D3, which is essential for building bone strength.

Use common sense when it comes to exposure to the sun. Sunscreen notwithstanding, limit your direct sun exposure to no more than ten minutes. If you've been exposed to direct sunlight for more than ten minutes on one day, give your skin a break and stay out of the blazing rays for the next couple of days.

"Days" are the time needed for your healthy skin cells to recover by replacing damaged cells and rebuilding protein structures in the skin.

People who have the habit of sun tanning cause their skin cells to get killed off and their protein structures to get damaged. Since they don't give the skin a break, there's no way any form of repair can take place effectively. The more they sit in the sun, the fewer healthy cells they have left. When this happens, the damage becomes permanent.

There is also that overhanging threat of skin cancer. Getting a tan not only causes your skin to age but is also a risk to your life.

Protect your skin from the sun using these measures:
- Women who wear make-up should use facial foundation with added sunblock.
- Use sunblock cream if you do not wear make-up.
- Protect your head if you have sparse hair or you're bald.
- If you have to spend a lot of time outdoors, wear enough material to cover your skin.

Remember, you can even be overexposed to UV rays when skies are overcast, so watch out.

Shielding the skin from UV damage is the most important skin-care measure you can take. Its effects will pay off. Sun-protected skin will look much healthier and better preserved in the long term.

Skin Abusing Substances to Avoid

Any substance that doesn't serve to feed the skin will ultimately damage it. While we cannot overly protect ourselves from the pollution in our environment, we can help ourselves by not adding more pollution to our skin.

Sources of skin-damaging substances we can reduce and avoid are the following:

- Chemicals from cigarette smoking
- Narcotics
- Prescription or over-the-counter drugs
- Allergens from food, cosmetics, or household products
- Sugar and alcohol
- Food additives

Skin is rich in blood. All kinds of chemicals get into the skin through the blood. Substances get locked up in skin tissue, some of which cause inflammation. Impurities build up in skin, and skin inflammation will damage natural skin structure.

As we age, skin gets more exposed to radiation, chemicals, and pollutants. This is partly the cause of skin deterioration. The best we can do for our skin is limit exposure to damage as much as we can by

- not smoking;
- staying clear of narcotics;
- saying no to unnecessary doses of medication;
- identifying allergens and avoiding them;
- reducing sugar and alcohol consumption; and
- eating whole foods instead of processed foods.

Your Skin Needs Food

Skin cells need to constantly metabolize, replenish, and build. They can achieve this only if they get enough of the essential nutrients necessary for healthy function.

Skin that gets fed with essential vitamins and minerals and that gets enough essential fatty acids and protein will glow with radiance.

If you really want good skin, spend less money on cosmetics and more money on quality food.

The only way to get nutrients to the skin cells is to eat well. A diet rich in nutrients and whole foods, and low in refined carbohydrates and alcohol, is great for the skin. You don't need to take expensive supplements. Getting your nutrients from your diet is the best way to get the right amounts and types of nutrients to your skin.

You don't need expensive skin creams and lotions. Contrary to marketing gimmicks, there is no way you can feed your skin from the outside. Skin gets nutrients only from blood.

Collagen is protein built by skin cells. Buying skin creams that contain collagen will not put collagen back into your skin. The only way to get collagen structures in the skin to grow back is to eat food high in protein and vitamins. Skin cells will receive the amino acids from the digested proteins through the bloodstream. In synergy with vitamins, minerals and hormones, rebuild the collagen structure in the skin.

Conversely, skin-care products that contain vitamins, amino acids, minerals, and even plant extracts do nothing to feed your skin. That just isn't possible. At best, you get the psychological effect of buying an expensive product. At worst, you get skin allergies from other chemicals in the cosmetics.

The only skin-care products worth buying are perhaps the following:

- Sunscreen
- Moisturizers
- Cleansers, scrubs, and freshening masks
- Mild exfoliating cleansers that contain alpha or beta hydroxy acids These are mild acids that make skin look smoother by helping dead outer layers of skin cells to drop off.

This isn't a very interesting collection, but you don't really need much more.

Keep it simple. The best skin solutions are often the simplest. The goal is all about protecting the skin from the outside, while feeding it from the inside. The simpler your skin regime, the more effective it will be. Nothing can replace good skin-care habits.

Cosmetic Surgery and other Aesthetic Procedures

The drawbacks of going to a cosmetic doctor are costs, downtime, pain, and risk. It is neither a good nor a bad idea. It is a personal choice. If you can afford the time and money for it, if you don't mind the drawbacks, *and* if it is the only thing that will make you feel better, it is probably justified.

Use only the services of reputed doctors. Your life is too valuable to save money on.

Choose procedures that are as noninvasive as possible. This means that if you have to choose between getting cut versus going with a milder procedure such as radio-frequency or laser treatment, choose the latter first.

Noninvasive treatments don't require incisions to the skin, though they may be uncomfortable or even painful. The most effective noninvasive procedures work by zapping away pigment and spots, scratching the surface to stimulate new cells to replace the old, and using radio-frequency waves to stimulate new collagen production.

Try not to get sold into doing more than you need. If a medical professional starts giving ideas about doing more than just lifting and smoothing, if he or she starts encouraging you to do more and more, or if you leave the consultation room feeling more lousy about your looks than before you arrived, you know you're being taken.

Cosmetic Procedures Cannot Make You Younger

Truth is, you can stretch, lift, pull, and polish your skin and still not have the image of youth. The procedure might help you look better in photos but not in person.

How often do we see movie stars who've had multiple expensive procedures look fabulously young in photos, only to look like old people with tightened skin in real life?

Also, cosmetic changes can make one feel a little more optimistic about his or her looks for a short period of time, but they are not a cure for poor self-image.

Body dysmorphia is a condition in which one obsesses over one's body imperfections. This obsession cannot be cured with cosmetic surgery. Self-hypnosis and therapy can help sufferers who, aware of their problem, are willing to get help.

Youth is really much more than skin deep.

If you do get procedures done, make them worth the money by working the process in synergy with the forever young, forever fit lifestyle. Only then will the skin heal properly and the effect last.

Effects of Stress on the Skin

The stresses and hardships of our lives show up in our faces. Observe the faces of people around you. As human beings get older, they display more of their life's issues on their faces.

Stress, as discussed in the previous chapter, is initiated in the mind. The brain sends out a cocktail of stress hormones that affect the physiology. While the entire body gets affected by stress, it is the skin that displays its effects most acutely.

The effects accumulate. Over time the lines, sagging, and spots on the skin deepen. Stress, a product of the mind, wreaks havoc on the skin. Relaxation can neutralize stress and the effects of stress. To relieve stress is to change the hormonal profile from a stressed state to a relaxed state.

We achieve this through relaxation techniques like meditation and self-hypnosis.

Skin Rejuvenation Meditation

Sit or lie down in a comfortable position. Breathe in and out slowly. Focus on that breathing and let your eye lids droop to a close.

Focus on every limb to relax the muscles until you feel like a limp rag doll.

Hold that pose and feeling. Focus on nothing but your breathing until your mind wanders nowhere.

If you're a beginner, your mind might return to thoughts that contain the stress. That is normal. When you become aware of this stress, relax and blank it out; focus on that breathing again.

Meditation, like everything in this book, is effective if you're able to make it a habit for life. Every time you meditate, you reset your mind. The relaxed mind produces a cocktail of hormones that are beneficial to the body for growth and rejuvenation.

For effective anti-aging of the skin, I have found one technique that can work for you:

In a relaxed state, let your mind travel back to a time of your childhood. Can you see the things around you? Maybe you're in school, kindergarten perhaps. Whose voice are you hearing? Could it be the voices of your friends? Could it be the voice of a teacher? How does the air feel? Are you indoors or outdoors? How does that air feel on the skin of your youthful face? How does that young skin feel? Can you feel the blood flowing under it, giving you a blush? Can you feel the sweat on that skin?

Hold that thought for as long as possible—perhaps about ten minutes.

Drift.

When you're ready, come back to the present. Open your eyes.

This method of meditation helps your skin remember what it was like to be young. Blood flows more efficiently, collagen is replenished, and skin firms up. Impurities will eventually fade because the relaxation halts the accumulation of stress.

The Hair Affair

Hair is like clothes in the sense that it is superficial elements of a person's look. One may have more flexibility with choice of clothes than with hair, since we each have our own hair types to work around. Your hair is an easy-to-manipulate personality statement. Its condition also gives an impression of your health and vitality.

Well-groomed, neatly kept hair is a generalized image of well-being. An ordered look indicates an ordered mind-set. It may not always be reality, but it is an impression.

"I wish I were taller and thinner but the hair you can do something about." Hillary Clinton

Make a statement with your hair

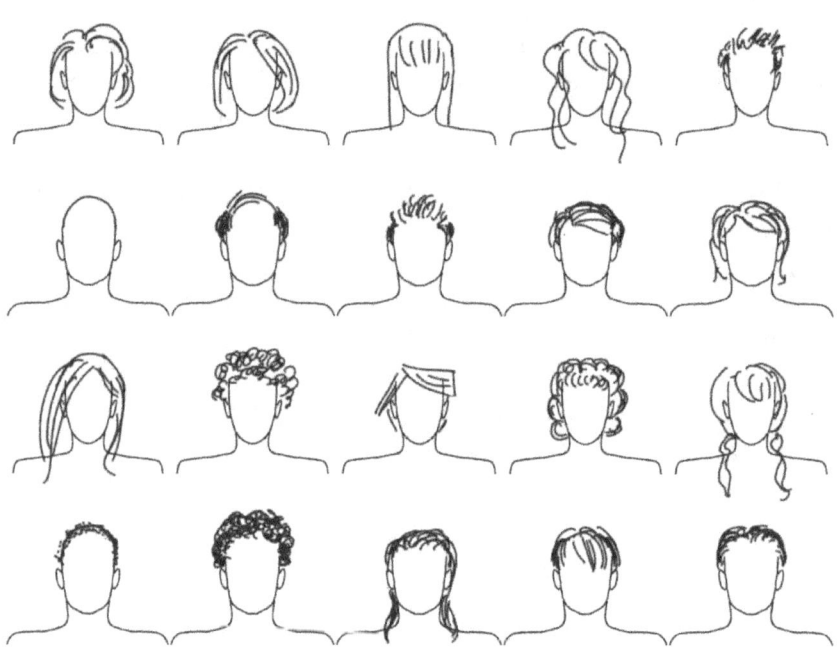

Order, as we discussed at the beginning of this book, is the state of health and youth. With order, even in our hair-styles, there is a greater possibility of looking more youthful.

We might argue that teenagers don't usually keep their hair neat, but that isn't the point. We shouldn't aim to look like teenagers; we should aim to look young and fit.

The idea that neat hair can make one look more youthful, however, has its exceptions. Some people really look better with messy hair. Feel free to explore the contemporary styles. Keep the look right by having hair you can manage. Fancy haircuts and coloring need constant touch-ups to keep the shape and color at the roots respectively. They are great fun to have if you have the time for regular trips to the salon.

Hair is dead material; overworking the hair with chemical treatments can cause it to look dull. It is best to put hair in as little contact as possible to perms, colors, and heat treatments. While there is really no such thing as "healthy hair," we can preserve luster and shine by protecting hair from damage.

A hairstyle is a display of one's fashion sense. As with clothes, one shouldn't stick to the same hairstyle for more than five years. Consider a general group of women born in the 1940s. How many of them still sport that "Jackie O" puffed-up hairdo? And women born in the 1960s—how many still wear hair from the eighties' punk rock movement? Change your look to keep from looking dated.

Men who are less inclined to experiment with new hairstyles should consider changing barber shop appointments for a makeover at a fashionable salon. Getting a fresh look every once in a while is good.

As we get older, hair issues, such as thinning and graying, tend to crop up. It is best to deal with these issues in a sensible way. Trying too hard to hide gray hair with outlandish hair color, wearing wigs that obviously look artificial, or tying to plaster hair over bald patches will have counter effects. Those are the things people tend to do with their hair to make themselves look ridiculously older.

If you have to cover up, make sure the job is done well; otherwise, embrace the situation. Bald is beautiful. Gray is divine.

While researching this section on hair, I stumbled upon articles on the Internet and in magazines that advise readers on the best hairdos to have according to age. This is like saying that there are approved hairstyles for ladies and men in their forties, while people in their sixties and seventies should wear their hair according to their "age." By age, they could mean only chronological age. Don't read them.

Wear your hair to look good, not to look like other people "your age."

As far as hair is concerned, change is refreshing. Try new styles. Use different stylists. When unsure, keep it simple and neat.

Fashion Statements

We want to look young and fit. A little more effort put into how we clothe ourselves can bring great dividends. Neglect for one's dress can make one look pretty much over the hill.

Dressing right is a habit that shouldn't be restricted to special occasions.

The fashion industry creates categories of fashion wear based on its market age-group. As we get older, we tend to gravitate toward styles that seem to suit our same-aged contemporaries. It could be because as we get older, we tend to take with us the fashion of our past. Fashion companies also create "older people fashion" to adapt to an older person's body shape. Hence there is such a thing as "old people fashion" and "young people fashion."

While it's great that companies are listening to their customers, the way they tailor clothes to fit people of different age groups, and the way the try to market these designs to us doesn't fit with our philosophy of being forever young and forever fit. How does one feel young when shopping at a granny fashion store? Definitely not like a young person.

By managing to stay fit by eating well and right, we should have a body shape that doesn't need special clothes adapted in shape to fit our bodies.

As advised in the previous segment on hair, the best advice for dressing right is to forget about "dressing your age."

Dress to look fabulous. Dress to express yourself. Dress to feel comfortable. Dress to move. Dress for success.

In general, clothes created for youth today tend to be shapelier, more "artistic," more open to variety of shape, design, and fabric. There is more experimentation. The clothes tend to be more affordable too. Be confident. Try them out. You might be surprised by how they bring out your looks.

Clothes created for the older generations tend to have bigger cuts, louder colors, baggy style, and less design variety. Some of these clothes might be beautiful, but you don't need to restrict your purchases in these stores.

Shop with an Open Mind

When it comes to buying clothes, be open minded. Choose variety. Shop everywhere.

If you have to pick a blouse from your favorite granny shop, pair it off with a scarf, belt, jacket, and stockings from the young people's fashion department.

Clothes that do not seem to go out of fashion, like denim wear. Slacks and shirts can be safe choices. Just remember that even these change in shape, tightness, and length with fashion trends.

It's not within the scope of this book to go into detail as to what makes dressing right. That kind of advice changes with time and varies with individual body shape, tone, and personality.

Cultivating a Dress Sense

Having a good dress sense can be cultivated if you take time to go shopping. Try on all kinds of clothes at the stores. Have a proper look at yourself and think, *Is this the look of the image I want?*

Remember that what you wear can affect how you feel about yourself. Clothes will affect the reality of how young you really are. Dress the way you like, not according to what the fashion industry or society dictates for people of your "age." They are talking about chronological age, and to us that is just a number.

Take some time off to be fashionable and try different types of clothes. Like dreams, trying out clothes in most stores is free. Never tell yourself, "I'm too old to wear this"—that is a myth and a limiting belief that fashion is age specific. A fashionable pair of slacks can look as good on a sixty-year-old as it would on a twenty-year-old.

The Hidden Dangers of Always Wearing Baggy Clothes

While wearing comfortable clothes that allow movement throughout the day is necessary, this doesn't mean we can go about town in frumpy pajama wear.

Baggy track suits, sweats, tent-like dresses, and so forth do have evil ways of making space between your skin and cloth to accommodate fatness.

Though there are exceptions, people who wear baggy clothes tend to get overweight without realizing it until it's too late.

Clothes can be the best gauge for your body fat percentage. If you're in the habit of wearing jeans that hug your hips and thighs, you will feel them straightaway if you put on even an eighth of an inch of fat on those areas. The jeans will become uncomfortable

In such a situation, you can do two things:
1.   Buy a bigger pair of jeans.
2.   Or don't buy a bigger pair of jeans and analyze your diet, exercise, and vow to get back into those jeans comfortably.

Choose the second option if you want to keep in shape. Buying clothes to make space for the extra flab is a bad idea.

Sloppy, baggy clothes are tricky for most of us to pull off. These will look disordered on our bodies. Disorder, as mentioned above, tends to create an impression of aging. If in doubt about choice of clothes, choose clean lines and simplicity. These keep the look "ordered" and will help most of us look younger.

Old Clothes Will Never Come Back In Fashion

Older folks I know never like throwing away anything. You don't really need to throw out your old clothes. Give them away to the poor.

Your closet should be clear of any clothing article that is more than a decade old—or five years old, if you can afford it. If you want to be sure you're really dressing right, keep no item of everyday wear for too long.

Clothes aren't like jewelry. Clothes don't get more valuable with time. They don't wear well when they are antiquated.

Why do younger people sometimes think people of their grandparents' generation dress funny?

Old people don't dress funny on purpose. Most of them simply never changed their wardrobe style since they were in their thirties. Decades pass, and they feel comfortable with their clothes. People identify them with their way of dressing. They don't feel comfortable changing their wardrobe.

Being aware of this is a reminder that you need to keep altering your style. A rolling stone gathers no moss. A changing style doesn't become antiquated. Old clothes don't really come back in fashion. One might argue that platform heels come back over and over again, but do they really?

If you have a habit of keeping old clothes, you'll just have the habit of wearing them. Eventually you'll look like everyone else in your age-group who has a similar attitude toward not changing his or her dress.

Ultimately nobody can look youthful by constantly wearing clothes that is decades old. Those who adopt the awareness are open minded in trying on new styles; they will outwit the rest and look forever young and fashionable.

What Lies on the Surface

That which seems superficial has deep roots that penetrate the inner self. Whatever is going on outside of us, like how our day has been, or how other people have made us feel, will affect our mood; and our moods affect how we act towards others. There is a kind of cycle of energy that flows from the superficial part of our being into our core and vice versa. This is not unlike the way a plant draws water and minerals from its roots to feed the leaves that absorb sunlight and provide energy back to the roots. How we look to the world will affect how the world reacts to us. This will in turn affect our emotions.

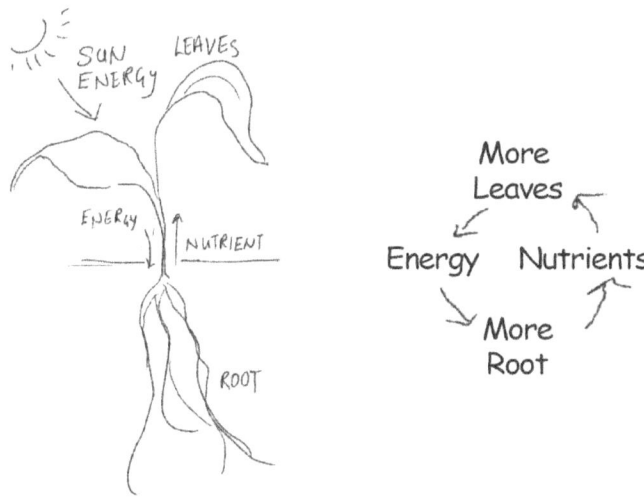

The brain stimulates a cocktail of hormones in response to emotions. Hormones activate cells, affecting our physiology. Depending on whether emotions are positive or negative, hormones can cause pleasure or stress. Positive emotions will bring better health than negative emotions.

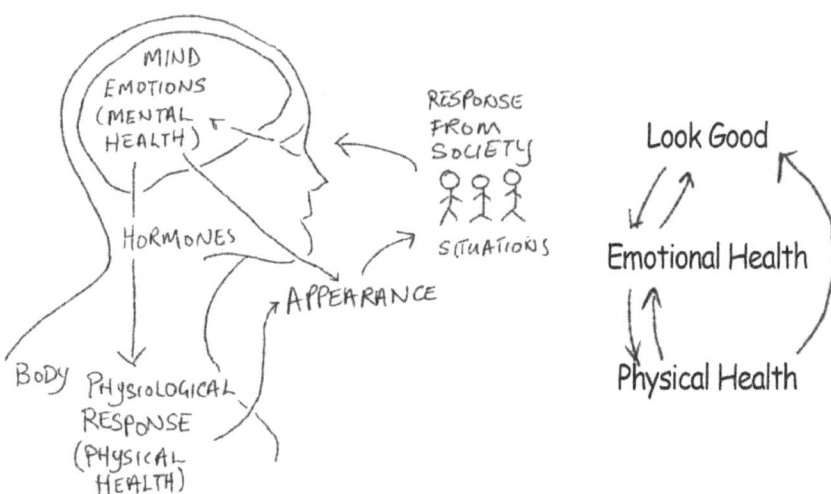

Physical appearance is a mirror of health. We can often judge someone's health or youth just by looking at his or her skin, posture, gait, voice, and so forth.

Emotional health affects physical appearance in two ways:

- By affecting the state of physical health
- By directly affecting physical appearance through actions such as dress, speech, attitudes, and so forth.

Since everything is a cycle, we can actually change the state of both mental and physical health by changing the way we look externally. We can do this by following some of the pointers in this chapter.

When you put effort into looking young, move with vigor, and dress in an ageless way, you exude vibrant youthfulness to the universe. Society will see that young person in you.

The world will regard your youthfulness and impart the energy to you that befits a young person.

You will feel that positive energy. This energy will register in your subconscious mind and affect your emotions. You will feel even more confident in your physical self.

A confident emotional state of mind stimulates the brain to produce hormones that bring pleasure to the body. This sets the whole body into a regenerative mode. You will find more energy available to you to live life to the full.

What the world sees in you is really what you get.

Chapter 8: What You Say is What You Get

The word is mighty.

Human dominance over all living creatures on this planet is founded on the word. We communicate our thoughts by stringing words together to form language. Communication allows us to impart lessons from life experiences down through generations.

Language is so powerful that it affects our minds in ways we aren't even aware of. Words used to tell a story in a novel or dramatic news heard on the radio can trigger emotional responses in us.

Mind and body, we know, are interconnected. When we listen to or read something, our minds analyze the words. Words stimulate our emotions. Emotions trigger hormonal responses, which affect our physiology.

The effects are observable signs like sweating and increased pulse when we read frightening news, or tears welling up when we read a sad novel. Our responses to these are rarely voluntary.

There are more subtle effects of language than outright fear or sadness. These effects are hardly noticeable to us.

We're constantly bombarded by words. We hear people talk. Things are communicated in the media, books, blogs, advertising, signs, and so on. These words affect our states of mind—our moods, emotions, and choices we make in life.

While words received passively affect how we are, the words we say or write etch our fate in stone.

Observe individuals around you and the kind of stuff they say or write, whether in passing or in all seriousness. Blogs and social media statuses are great places to observe other people's language.

People often repeat themselves, and their words are a reflection of their personalities. What they say often reflects how they really are and the situation they are in.

Complaining about the same things over and over will not make things better. Things usually deteriorate more quickly with people who spend their lives lamenting. If we substitute our urge to complain with affirmations for positive change, things will improve. The little improvements will snowball into significant progress.

This is true for every aspect of our lives, not just in health and fitness.

The reverse is also true. What we say actually makes us who we are. How we talk about our situations in life manifests into full-blown reality.

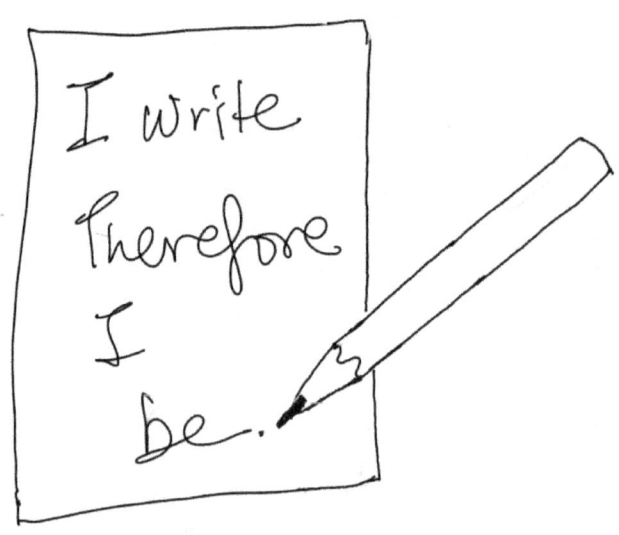

What we say is what we will get eventually.

Look back at everything you have said or written. What do your words reflect? Do they reflect a positive state or a negative state of life?

If it is true that words can change our lives, wouldn't it be worthwhile to try changing all negative words into positive messages?

How do we use language to stay forever young and forever fit?

Words and the Subconscious Mind

The human mind is made up of two compartments of thought. One is the conscious mind, the thoughts we control, like our daily thoughts, decisions, and so forth. The other part, the subconscious mind, is like a hard disk that secretly absorbs peripheral information and stores it in our memory.

The study of language's effect on the subconscious mind has become an exact science. Some call it neurolinguistic programming or NLP. It is a concept that has been understood for decades and used for psychotherapy, hypnosis, and even marketing.

Words have influence over the subconscious mind. The subconscious mind is the part of our awareness we're least able to control. Sometimes our subconscious minds picks up and store messages we aren't even aware of.

There's a link between our subconscious minds and our bodies. The subconscious mind, when filled with thoughts of youthfulness, fitness, relaxation, and positivity, will lead us to a life in the positive direction. The opposite is also true. Be aware of your daily words, because your subconscious mind picks them up and transforms them into reality. Such is the power of words.

The Language of Vitality

Always talk yourself healthy.

"I am fit and healthy." We don't hear people say this about themselves enough.

Instead, we hear, "Oh, I got a headache" or "Spring is here, and I got allergies."

Many would post or tweet every ache, pain, and allergy attack on social media. For some reason, complaining about illnesses attracts more attention. Attention, usually in the form of well wishes and sympathy, acts as a reward for those who seek it.

The danger of getting rewarded for proclaiming ill health is *getting* persistent ill health. Subconsciously, we get hooked on feelings of reward, regardless of where they originate.

On days when you feel under the weather, try not to talk unnecessarily about how sick you feel unless it is with your doctor. Try not to wear sickness as a badge, sharing it with everyone you meet.

Don't habitually write about illnesses, aches, and pains online. Keep all tweets on a positive, self-fulfilling note.

If you really need to talk about an episode of ill health, you would be best to wait till you have fully recovered. Go ahead and tell the world how you overcame the illness. The world will benefit from the means you took to get yourself well again. Recommend the doctor or therapist who helped you.

The same principle applies for proclamations of anything negative—depression, bad news, scary news, paranoia, and so forth.

Saying nothing is better than putting anything negative in the written word, because what you say is what you will eventually get.

Harp on sickness, and you will find yourself sniffing a lot. Say you're depressed, and the depression will stick.

Experiment with talking in positives. You might find this to be a simple, life-changing habit.

Talking positively will make your life better. Positive words bring luck, happiness, and good health.

Being positive is like the analogy of looking at a glass that is half empty or half full.

Talking positively is easier than thinking positively. Positive thinking can be a strain. Negative thoughts, doubts, dislikes, envies, insecurities, and so on tend to be attached to emotions. They can be hard to shake off.

The good news is that talking positively is as beneficial as thinking positively. If your thoughts are negative, say something positive. Write something positive. Things will gradually change for the positive.

Some call this the power of attraction.

The power of attraction is the idea that everything you say, write, do, and preoccupy your thoughts with will eventually manifest in your life.

For example, if you want to stay fit and healthy, think fit and healthy. It's better to do stuff that makes you fit and healthy. Read books like this one to stay fit and healthy. You have a better chance of reaching your goals by doing positive things than by complaining about getting old or having no time to exercise or even saying, "I don't want to get old."

Talk is not cheap. It's an action that can manifest into reality. If you're so utterly depressed that you can't summon the strength to write or say something positive, say nothing and do things like these:

- Meditate.

- Do something physical like exercise or dance.

- Go to sleep.

- Take a long warm shower.

- Engage in a hobby.

The best you can do when you feel chronically depressed is to seek the help of others. Isn't that after all what we are here for; to help and be helped?

You can also turn aside setbacks by setting goals, vocalizing these goals, and making a plan on how to make things work.

The Written Word is Also the Word

The written word is actually much more potent than the spoken word. Why? While the spoken word is sound, the written word is taken in as sight. Light travels much more quickly than sound. Therefore, words we read get into our brains much more clearly and quickly than the stuff we hear.

Writing negative and self-defeating things online is akin to carving your fate in stone.

No matter how crappy your day has been or how sick and old you feel or how inadequate you feel trying to catch up with a younger person, don't write about it. Don't even write it in an e-mail to your closest friend or post it on social media.

Strategize instead on getting fitter and stronger, focus on your progress, and put those gains into words. Share your successes with everyone. This way you'll benefit from the power of your own words. You'll inspire others to do well. The world will be a better place.

While you're on social media, blogging and e-mailing, write words of encouragement and youthfulness. Praise other people's gains and successes. When you give support, you get support back. Support from others can go a long way to helping you achieve your own goals.

Share your personal health tips. Encourage others to take on a positive, healthy mind-set.

You, in turn, will benefit from your own words.

Support Others with Encouraging Words

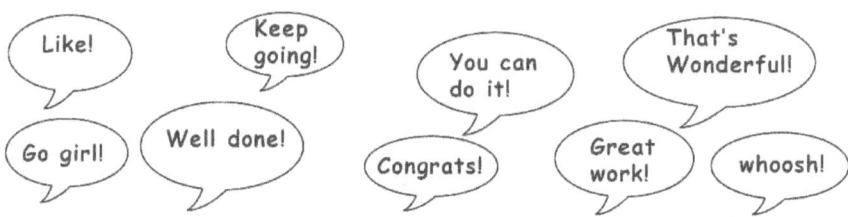

Some Things Never to Say to Yourself

We often unknowingly make ourselves old by our words. Sometimes our disdain for getting old leads us into identifying ourselves as old people.

Depending on our personalities, we talk ourselves down because of several reasons:

- We want someone to negate our comment and say instead, "No, you're not old."

- We're trying to tell ourselves it's OK to get old because it's normal and because everyone gets old anyway.

- We wish to find something positive about being old, such as the benefits of being a senior citizen or the idea that "we get older and wiser."

The problem is that the more we talk ourselves down, the worse off we get. This becomes a vicious cycle.

Here are just some of the phrases we should refrain from saying:

"I'm too old for..."

This is an excuse not to do something. If we don't want to do or learn something, we use age as an excuse. The older we get, the easier it is to get out of doing something by saying, "I'm too old for..." In the process, we tell ourselves we're too old to do stuff. This will not make us younger because the subconscious mind hears us say, "I'm too old..." Our words become a self-fulfilling prophecy.

"At my age..."

Similar to the earlier phrase, we use this as an excuse not to do things.

"It is not possible now that I am x years old."

Every year you get older, you wear a badge? Celebrate that now you're not going to do this and this and this. Eventually your subconscious mind decides that doing even more isn't possible, and your body responds by taking away your ability to do things.

"I'll leave it to the young people."

When you say, "I'll leave it to the young people," you're thinking that you're not young yourself. You undermine your state of youth. If you want to be forever young and forever fit, *you* are the "young people." Therefore, that statement will not make sense.

"Young people nowadays..."

Like the earlier statement, if you criticize "young people" in general, you're omitting yourself from the youth group. This statement doesn't hurt the people you're critiquing; it only hurts yourself.

"The music was better when I was young."

Oh, come on! That is absolutely untrue. The past is full of good things and also full of crap. The attitude of forever young and forever fit is to adopt open-mindedness.

Learn to Ignore Other People's Negative Writing

Once we're aware of the effects of words on our psyche, we can learn to ignore negative messages others have posted.

Written words tend to hold the most weight. Learn to differentiate between facts and casual remarks. Ignore negative talk and limiting beliefs. Don't take what others say personally.

Things printed on paper can often be tossed in the trash. Words posted on the Internet can disappear with one click.

If you find other people's trivial comments difficult to ignore, be quiet, meditate, listen to music, dance; do anything to clear your mind of disturbances.

"Smilers never lose and frowners never win."

Lyrics from the song, "Open Up Your Heart (And Let The Sun Shine In)"

Talk Yourself Young

Words can change your body. You can talk yourself young. Listen to the chatter around you and notice the difference between the vocabulary of youthful people and old people. People who look better and younger just talk differently from everyone else. This may sound like a generalization, but we can observe some of these attributes:

- They have more positive things to say about new developments in their society. It could be a new technology, fashion, music, and so forth.
- They talk well about their state of health.
- They talk with optimism about their immediate future. They have plans.
- They always encourage others to try new things.
- They are inspirational.
- They are never afraid to praise themselves.
- They share ideas and give out compliments.
- They listen.
- They seek help when they need help.

Some of these behaviors may seem lacking in humility or sound a bit egotistical, but talking humbly or self-critically to gain other people's favor is insincere and serves only to hurt the self.

Besides, true friends will be happy only when they say you're OK.

Taking control of the words you use in writing and in speech is not a big task. Like everything else mentioned in this book, it is a habit to cultivate and turn into a lifestyle.

The best thing about being positive with your words is that this is an easy habit to adopt. The changes you can make with this new awareness can be outstanding—small changes that brings great rewards.

Chapter 9: A Timeless Mind-Set

To be forever young and forever fit, one has to think forever young and forever fit.

Every manifestation of success (or failure) has its origins in our minds.

Thinking young and fit will lead us to being young and fit. Any other way would be impossible.

Going through the motions of exercising, dieting, dressing young, or even getting cosmetic surgery would be fruitless if one had the wrong mind-set.

Thinking we're old is the number one cause of aging. For most of us, this begins very early in life. We allow society to define us by our age.

It starts when we're kids; the adults in our lives celebrate our "growing up." Then when we're teenagers, they celebrate us "being grown up." Then when we become parents, workers, and employers, we celebrate our importance as matured individuals.

Up to that point, life seems like a celebration. Unfortunately that process doesn't end right there.

When we reach our forties, society tells us we're middle aged, which means we're categorically not young people anymore. By our sixties, society considers us old, and by our eighties we're considered aged. By the time we approach one hundred, they count every year we stay alive and celebrate it like it's something out of the ordinary.

When we allow others to identify us by our chronological age, we subconsciously identify ourselves that way too.

When we think of ourselves as getting older, we play the role of the older person. We allow society to put us in an age box. To stay forever young and forever fit, we need to get ourselves out of the box. Before we can get ourselves out of the box, we must believe that it exists and know what it looks like.

"You know someone said the world's a stage, and each must play a part..." That's from the lyrics to the song "Are You Lonesome Tonight?" sung by Elvis Presley; the lyrics are derived from a Shakespearean quote.

The world's a stage, *but* we should decide for ourselves what we want to do on it.

Simplistic ideas like classifying people according to their age-group, sex, ethnicity, and so forth are limiting beliefs. Limiting beliefs ingrained in our minds stop us from clarity of thought. Very often these beliefs hinder personal progress while keeping us in a depressed state of mind.

The best way to sever ourselves from limiting beliefs is to become fully aware of their existence in the first place.

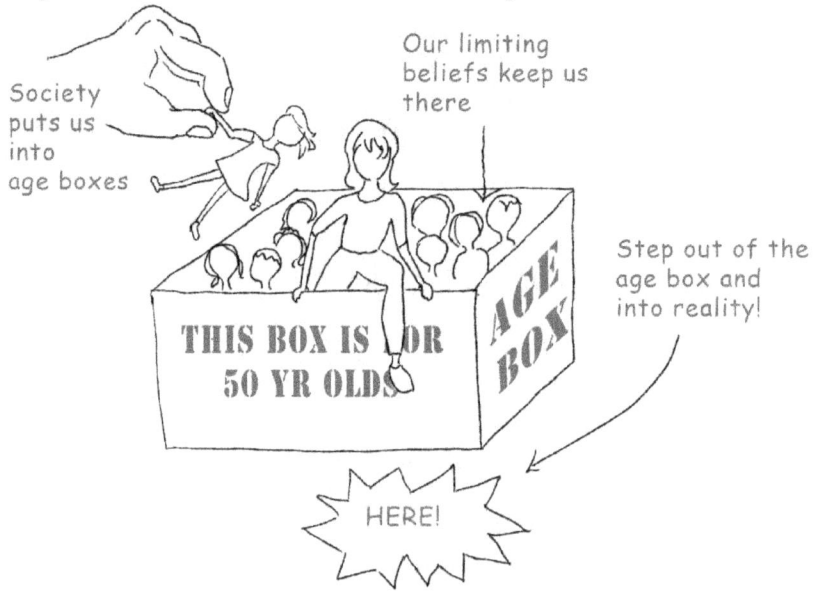

Society puts us into age boxes

Our limiting beliefs keep us there

THIS BOX IS FOR 50 YR OLDS

AGE BOX

Step out of the age box and into reality!

HERE!

Things Only Get Better

Optimism makes us young. When the mind thinks well of the future, the body prepares itself for something good to happen.

Believe in the goodness of the human spirit. Things will only get better. Humanity has progressed so far for general good. Seek not the old days, be they bad or good.

The past is past and has ceased to exist. The only existence of past events is in our memories. We don't need to forget the past, but we need to learn not to live in it.

Living in the past will cause us to get stuck in the past. Getting stuck in the past stunts our mental development. It causes us to lose track of time, lose interest in society, and lose touch of what's happening in the world. Losing touch leads to loss, which equals aging.

Keep your mind young by keeping yourself abreast with the present world.

To live in the now is to enjoy the journey—the purring of the car, the music on the stereo, the passing landscape. Life is a journey made enjoyable when there is no fixation on where you have come from, which is the past, or your destination, which is the future.

Embrace Development

Having an open mind is instrumental to mental growth. Growth builds. Take interest in new things: new gadgets, new cuisines, new fashion, new music, new people, and so on.

Young people generally accept change and embrace development more readily than old people do. There is a tendency for us to cling to things of the past while rejecting anything that seems unfamiliar. We do this because familiarity is our comfort zone. The older we get, the more we seem to need comfort.

Accept new development and let go of the past. This will keep you current. You will remain socially viable, able to interact with people of all ages without suffering the "generation gap."

Never let your thoughts tell you they made better music when you were young. That is a limiting belief, not reality. People make good and bad music, no matter which era it is. If you think music of the past was better, that's only because you've ceased to listen to the new stuff and accept it. You've not learned to appreciate the development of music. In this aspect, you've got yourself musically stuck in the past.

You might think, *How does something so basic as appreciating the latest pop hits become such a big deal?*

Spin this further to everything else in life. You may find yourself gradually losing touch with many other things besides pop music. How often do you hear of somebody's grandparents not being able to handle a simple mobile phone or the ATM?

How do old people get from being vibrant working adults to being excluded from society?

Unless there's sudden illness or disability involved—and that's not even a good reason to fall back—people don't lose touch with the world from one day to the next. It happens insidiously with the little things, like saying, "They wrote better songs in the good old days" or "I'm too old to learn."

Learn, explore, and be curious. Embrace all kinds of change. Stay young.

The Time Traps

We're all individual beings. We're not actually what we identify ourselves superficially with. We're not even our names, because if we changed our names tomorrow, we would remain who we are.

Family, possessions, societal responsibilities, obligations, roles, and so forth are all external things we unwittingly identify ourselves with. We often say, "My children," "My parents," "My jobs," "My possessions," "My successes," "My thoughts," "My intelligence"— almost anything and everything that relates to us—while attaching all these external projections to our own identity.

This holds true for every other thing we attach our identities to. It could be "I am Jackie's mother" or "I am a CEO of GM CORP" or "This is my Porsche" or "I am a renowned artist" or "I am a handicapped veteran."

What happens if we say, "I am," and add nothing else? Saying just "I am" might feel somewhat strange.

When we mistake these projections in our lives for our personal selves, we make ourselves vulnerable. Projections are like extra limbs. They are temporal and very susceptible to damage. We feel the pain when these limbs get injured, damaged, or even chopped off.

Detaching our sense of self from these projections can save us from unnecessary suffering. We can still control the life around us "wirelessly" with a remote control. Things will still function as well, if not better. When they cease to be of use or when these things get destroyed, we don't get hurt along with them.

Everything we attach our identities to eventually become time traps. These attachments change, and some get damaged with time. For example, our roles change when the kids grow up. Our jobs change or disappear; cars go out of fashion; our looks change; our beliefs change.

When we're able to separate our sense of identity from the world around us, we enjoy life even more. When change happens, we don't get a shock or feel depressed because we expect everything to be as it was in the past.

Understanding this philosophy brings clarity. Being able to see things with clarity makes us better able to adapt to change.

What significance does this fact have on the aging state of mind?

It can be observed when parents say they "feel old" upon seeing their children grow up. This is an example of an external factor evoking the feeling of being old. Remember that when the mind feels something, the body usually reacts to that feeling by being that feeling.

Hence, witnessing children grow up leads to feeling old, which leads to actually getting old.

When we let go of identifying ourselves with the role of parent, we can enjoy children as individuals—individuals who will grow and change. We're better able to accept the fact of our children growing up and the world changing around us without attaching this change to the idea that we're growing old along with the change.

There are many examples in life that will make us feel the passage of time—for example, retirement, death in the family, children leaving home, the coming of grandchildren, the leaving of friends, and the change in society. These changes become time traps when we attach ourselves too tightly to them.

Free yourself of these time traps. Let go of the need to identify yourself with external things, no matter how dear they are to you. When you can free yourself of these attachments, you can enjoy your family, job, money, stuff, role, achievements, and so forth as you always did and much more. The only difference is that when these transient things change, you're better able to embrace the change and not suffer the loss by clinging to the past.

Find time in your busy schedule to meditate on what it means to be you—just you.

Take time to relax and clear your mind from external disturbances.

Try to think about what the phrase "I am" actually means—just "I am" and not "I am ___."

Try to understand what "I am" means without any word coming after it.

Feel the sense of being. That being has no role, no superficial identity, and no possessions because it is timeless. Being timeless is being ageless. It can be a very liberating experience.

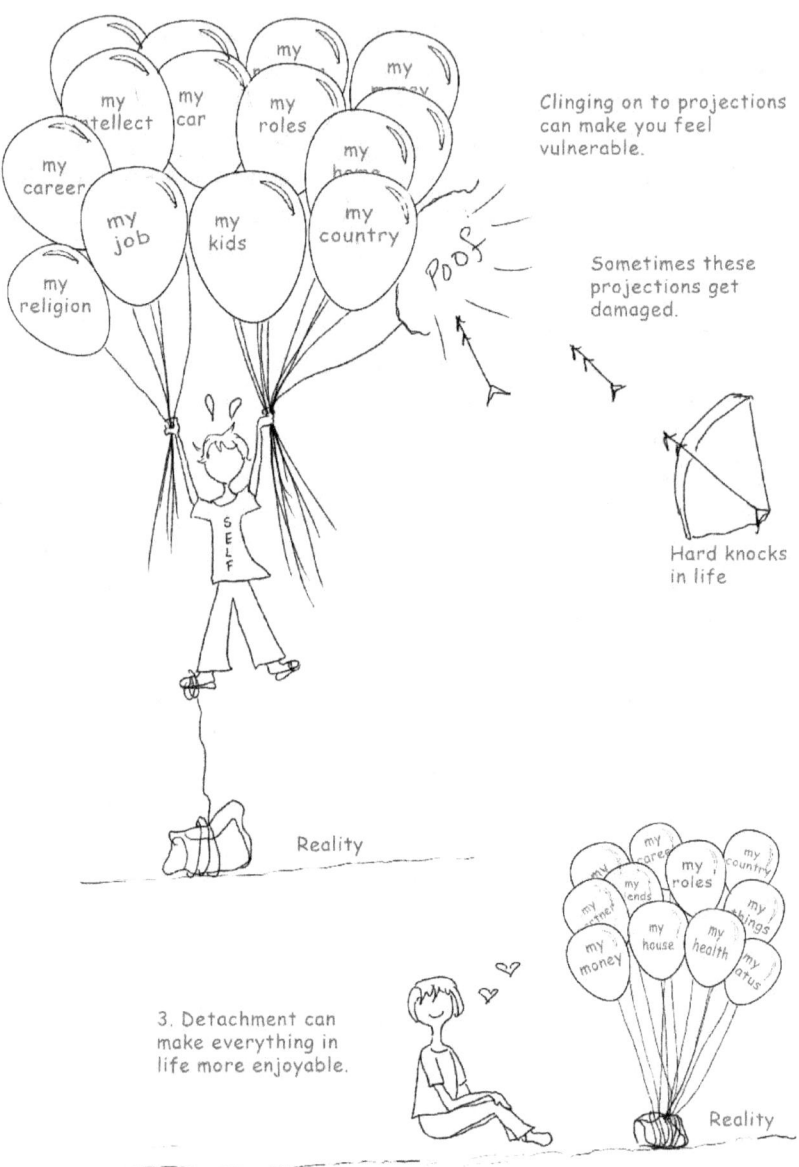

Clinging on to projections can make you feel vulnerable.

Sometimes these projections get damaged.

Hard knocks in life

Reality

3. Detachment can make everything in life more enjoyable.

Reality

Life Goes On—Meditation

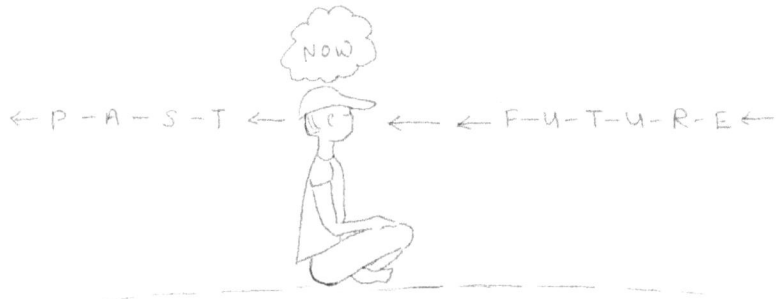

An empowering way to meditate is to visualize the self as a stationary force. Sit relaxed and take time to imagine that you're absolutely still, while the passage of time passes through you.

Feel the past behind you. You're facing the future. The future is coming toward you. The future touches you, and the future becomes the present. The present moves on to the back of you, becoming the past.

A new present touches you.

You're living in the present. You're always living in the present. There is no other reality.

The world moves toward you, through you, and behind you. You're still you. That is the feeling of timelessness.

We don't have full control of our fates, but we have power over how we see ourselves in life situations.

We can develop in ourselves a sense of being that keeps us in a reality of the present. When we're in the present, we cannot live in the past at the same time. When we live in the present, everything is a new beginning, a new experience, a new awakening. There is no time for feeling old or getting old. There is only the promise of feeling forever young.

"Nobody can go back and start a new beginning, but anyone can start today and make a new ending." Maria Robinson

Chapter 10: Beat Your Own Drum

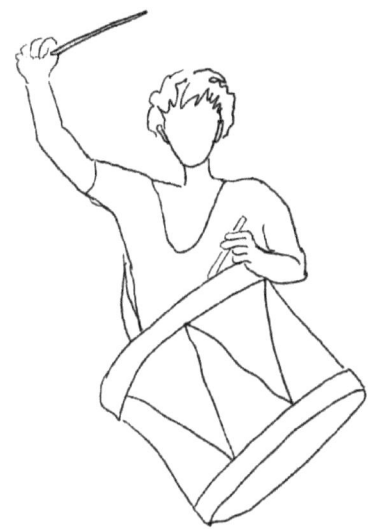

Aging and ageism are uniquely human concepts. We're all programmed to get old. By late adulthood, we start to do less, we start to dress and talk differently, we use our age as an excuse for things, and we think of retirement.

This programming is attributed to our ability to communicate. As a society we collectively decide to get old, slow down, retire, and even die when we reach milestones of our chronological age.

We have discussed how society puts us in age boxes. We get put in our age boxes from the very day we're born. Society expects everybody to be the same when he or she reaches a certain chronological age.

Society treats people not as individuals. We cannot see Mabel as Mabel but as a preschooler. We don't see Andy as Andy but as Mabel's dad. We don't see Susan as Susan but as Mabel's grandaunt.

As we discussed in the previous chapter, age is just one of many projections in our lives by which we identify ourselves and others.

Projections are labels. Labels are great for handbags, because depending on the brand inscribed on the label, they increase the value of the merchandise.

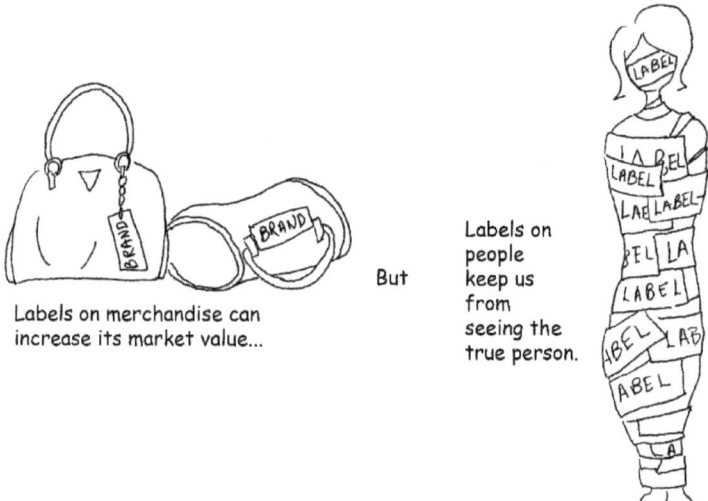

Labels on merchandise can increase its market value...

But

Labels on people keep us from seeing the true person.

But human beings are not merchandise.

Putting labels on people only serves to diminish the true value and greatness of the individual.

Separating oneself and others from their labels is not difficult to do. Like everything that needs to be done for a change in lifestyle, being aware that these labels exist is a great starting point.

The questions to ponder are:

Who are we, really? When we meditate on this question, we will realize there is an infinite power behind the self.

Do we like the labels society puts on us? Perhaps we do. Some labels we're proud of, while others we may not like at all.

What happens when these labels crack? Do we crack with them? The truth is that we often do crack if the labels we live off are damaged. For example, many people suffer depression on retirement, because they cannot let go of being identified with their role in society while working for a company.

Most of these labels actually act to conceal our real potential from the rest of the world.

Labels that evoke negative emotions can be let go of. That is good news as long as we're aware of their existence.

Do we put labels on others in efforts to identify ourselves? We often do, and thus we need to be careful of this, since putting labels on others is evidence of a limiting belief waiting to impose on our own happiness.

When we're aware of labels and let go of them, we expose our unique and special selves. Each of us is capable of creativity, a potential in every human spirit to be truly great.

Each of us has a drum to beat. It is like the heartbeat of the soul. The less we allow society to direct our sound, the more we're able to realize our true rhythm.

Change Can Actually Be a Lonely Thing

If you're someone who feels the need to have support from the people around for everything you do, you may find making lifestyle changes almost impossible to achieve if nobody else around shares your vision.

Often when we try to make these changes, the biggest resistance comes from those closest to us: the folks at home, friends, and the people at work.

We have all had our share of trying to encourage close friends and family to make healthy choices. It's not easy. The resistance is ever present.

As mentioned in the foreword of this book, I faced resistance too, but I learned very quickly the value of going my own way and taking the lead.

"Do just once what others say you can't do, and you will never pay attention to their limitations again." James Cook

Take the Lead

Taking the lead in life situations isn't everybody's cup of tea. Some people are more dependent on others, and some need community support and approval to do things, while others go about things on their own steam.

You take full control of your well-being. The world can provide support, but responsibility rests on your willingness to make things happen. You owe it to yourself, as well as everyone who depends on you, to feel good and look great.

Being healthy, fit, and current benefits the self and the community around the self. Everyone will benefit from your success in leading a forever young, forever fit lifestyle, even if he or she didn't provide support.

By staying young and fit, you
- live a productive life for as long as possible;
- have the capacity to care for others;
- are a shining example to your community;
- are living life to the full, making best use of your divine gifts;
- don't drain the resources of others;
- stay valuable to society; and
- feel great for yourself.
    Eventually your success will inspire even the hardest cynic.
To those in your life who will never accept your resolve, let them be.

Time For Yourself

Set a timetable from your daily schedule to include time for yourself. You need time for the following:
- Exercise. Always make time for a workout. You just need thirty minutes.
- Meditation. This is time for relaxation. You need time to de-stress. Take the most convenient time off for meditation. It could be the hour after you wake up or time after your workout.
- Sleep. Nothing is more important than sleep. Guard that time and don't allow anyone to deprive you of the body-regenerating function of sleep.
    Claim your own time. Make others understand they need to respect that time you set for yourself.

The Real Diet Challenge

Since you're fully aware that eating french fries with sugary ketchup will make you physically ill, you don't ever have to eat it. Even if
- your spouse insists on eating french fries with ketchup at every meal;
- your teenage kids insist on eating french fries with ketchup at every meal;

- your dominating aging parent insists on eating french fries with ketchup at every meal; or
- your colleagues insist on french fries at eat-ins during those long office meetings.

You should never feel compelled to eat what everybody else eats.

Put healthy options in your kitchen or office and eat them yourself if others insist on eating junk.

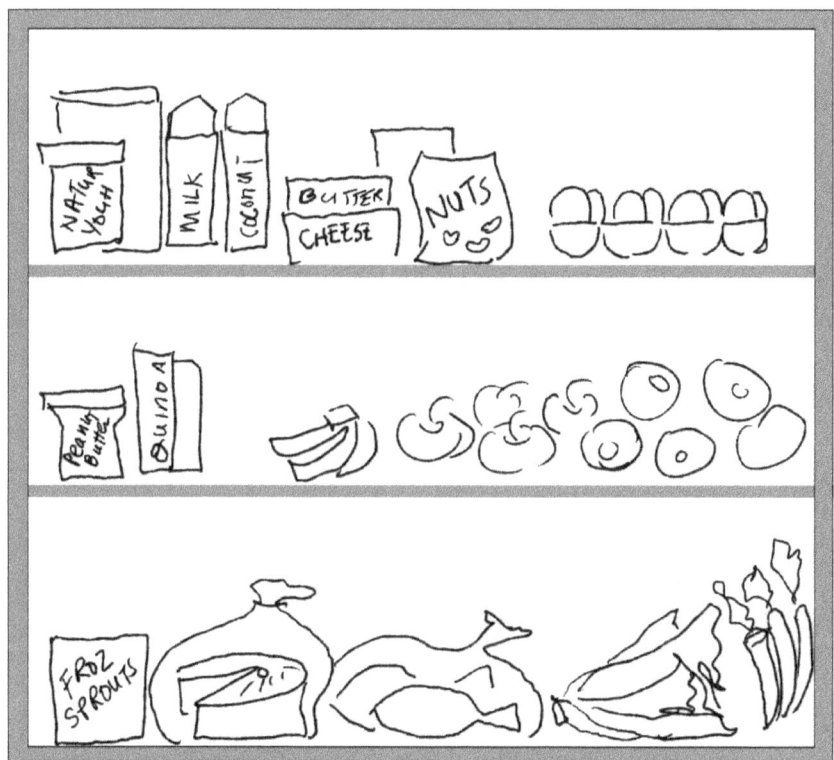

Stock Your Shelves with Good Food

Other people's junk food lying around the house or the office may undo your resolve to eat clean.

What will help is allocating your own shelf space in the kitchen cabinet and refrigerator and only eating food kept in those areas.

If you're responsible for the cooking, cook larger portions of healthy food and less of the junk food that the rest prefer to eat. Learning to cook well can also help the rest of the family wean off poor food choices.

The real diet challenge is not knowing what to eat, knowing how to cook, or having the willpower to make changes to your daily meals. The real diet challenge is dodging junk food put in front of you by those who are well meaning or ignorant or who couldn't care less.

Share this book. It was purposefully written to keep things simple for members of your family to read and hopefully enjoy. It will help them understand the concepts and benefits of a healthy lifestyle so you can all support each other on your quest to keep your diet clean.

Listen for the beat of your own drum!

Freedom to make a lifestyle change is your right. Create your own life's rhythm. Motivate yourself.

Honor Your Principles

Every individual lives with good intentions. Each of us, however, has his or her own set of values. Each of us has a unique set of rules to live by. The rules we make for ourselves actually put us on a course that make us feel secure.

Treasure your own principles. You don't need to compromise them at the whim of others. People who care for you will respect your principles.

By now, you will already have an idea of what you need to change to stay forever young and forever fit. Write in a diary a set of resolutions you know will help you achieve your goals.

Set your own goals.

Use this book as a guide. Set a road map of goals for the short and medium term so that the big picture is one of success.

Set your workout schedule, have a food diary, make time for meditation, set new sleeping hours, get a closet overhaul. These make up tiny little goals you can achieve.

The key to getting things done is to set your own goals. You can choose to follow other people's programs, but that wouldn't be enough without targets. Doing something without a clear goal is like going on a trip without knowing the destination.

The desire, planning, and execution are entirely up to you. With the knowledge gathered from the pages of this book, you can better assess some of the really good programs available online and offline. These are the pathways available for you to reach your goal.

The goals you set for yourself should be doable, but they should also be challenging.

There are no shortcuts to any place worth going to.

The less time you give yourself for overcoming a hurdle, the more success you will achieve, and the more inspired you will be to keep going.

When you're able to achieve the goals you set for yourself, when you see progress, when you become an inspiration to yourself, you beat your own drum. Enjoy the rhythm.

Practice makes perfect. After a while, you will find your rhythm. This new lifestyle will become second nature. It will become effortless.

Staying forever young and forever fit will become a reality—for you.

Congratulate Yourself

Every time you overcome a hurdle in your life, congratulate yourself. You don't need to hold a party. All you have to do is to say, "Well done!"

When you're able to acknowledge your success and vocalize it, more success will come to you. That is the time for you to spread that rhythm to the rest of the world.

You will get healthier. You will look younger. You will feel more confident and energetic. People will notice that positive change in you. Society will react to the fresh you by sending you positive feedback. I wish you a lifetime of feeling great, confident, and sexy—all the positive emotions that lead to a healthy life.

A Final Note

Finishing the last chapters of this book, I realized that in midst of the excitement, I forgot lunch. You know how it is, the sudden realization of hunger. I go to the kitchen, and a stockpile of Christmas goodies beckons. It is the season for merry-making and, you know, we have to enjoy our special occasions, so I dug in like Cookie Monster from Sesame Street. It is alright to fall off the wagon every once in a while; as long as you *know* you have fallen off the wagon.

Living forever young, forever fit is a flexible lifestyle choice. There are goals to make. These goals are based on rules to follow. These rules arise out of the awareness of what is necessary for positive change. I am a firm believer that awareness alone is the start to solving all the issues we face in life.

Bringing awareness is the true message of this book. I hope these chapters will enhance your interest in taking better care of your health, and that you'd be inspired to learn more about topics mentioned here. When faced with lifestyle choices, you will know the right ones to make.

If this book has been a benefit to you, share it. Spread the message. Share the gift of being forever young, forever fit.

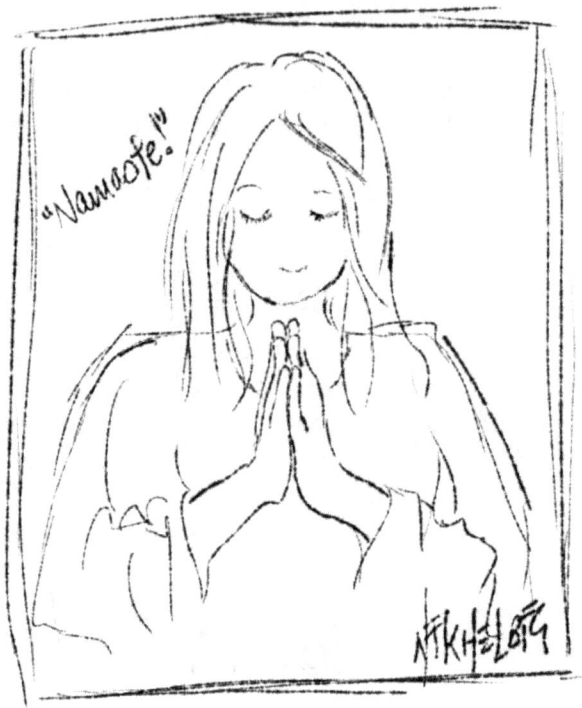

ABOUT THE AUTHOR

Nik Helbig started her career as a biochemist for the food and medical industries. In the last decade, she has extended her work towards the more practical aspect of the sciences by helping others to understand the fundamentals of health and fitness. The road to guiding others has encouraged her to reach deeper into studies in neurolinguistic programming or NLP, Enneagram research, and methods of self-hypnosis and meditation. The combined effect of knowledge in these fields has proven to be tremendously useful to her clients, many of whom are business professionals from Asia and the EU. When not at work (or working out), Nik indulges in painting, traveling and of course, shopping.

www.ingramcontent.com/pod-product-compliance
Lightning Source LLC
Chambersburg PA
CBHW070648290526
45790CB00001B/229